OUTSIDE THE LINES

... of love, life, and cancer

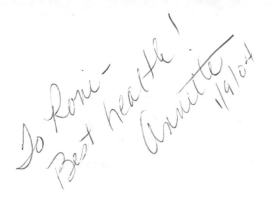

To Roni –
Best health!
Annette 1/9/04

OUTSIDE THE LINES

... of love, life, and cancer

This is a true story of empowerment
during catastrophic illness.

Annette Leal Mattern

Annette Leal Mattern

Skyward Publishing, Inc.
Dallas, Texas
www.skywardpublishing.com

Publisher: Skyward Publishing, Inc.
               17440 N. Dallas Parkway, Suite 111
               Dallas, Texas 75287
               (972) 490-8988
               E-mail: info@skywardpublishing.com
               Website: www.skywardpublishing.com

Library of Congress Cataloging-In-Publication Data

Mattern, Annette Leal, 1949-
    Outside the lines : of love, life, and cancer : this is a
true story of empowerment during catastrophic
illness / Annette Leal Mattern.
        p. cm.
    ISBN 1-881554-33-3
1. Mattern, Annette Leal, 1949---Health.
2. Ovarian--Cancer--Patients--Oregon--Biography. I. Title.
RC280.P25 M38 2003
362.1'9699437'0092--dc21

                                    2003011775

Printed in the United States of America.
Cover Design by Angela Underwood
Illustrations by Annette Leal Mattern

*For my beloved husband, Rich, who turned
a long night's journey into day.*

When we were kids, Mother never let us have coloring books. She said they were bad for us because they taught us to only see that which is inside the lines.

"You don't need anyone telling you how or where you should color," she would say. "Go outside the lines."

Table of Contents

From My Beginning

Ours was not a happy childhood growing up in South Texas, largely because Daddy was an abusive alcoholic who couldn't keep a job and was not above gambling away his occasional paycheck or the family car. There were many times, too many, really, when arguments with Mother got out of hand. As kids, my two sisters, Carmen and Sylvia, and I always had to be on guard, never knowing when an eruption would occur. And, more than once, I secretly wished that he would die.

We were a poor family. Mother taught third grade across town in a Mexican neighborhood and earned a modest salary. We lived in a two-bedroom house across the street from the railroad tracks, a shack, really, as I look back on it. Although Mother tried to manage all of our needs, Daddy's drinking and carousing and drifting from job to job left us always on the brink of one crisis or another as far back as I can remember:

"Yes, I know the bill's overdue, but you can't turn off our heat."

"What do you mean, he's in jail?"

"We're leaving, girls. Get in the car—right now."

There were many hardships. And although the scars are very deep, I believe that ultimately those hardships made us resourceful. And Mother, for all her mistakes or misjudgments, passed along to us a strong work ethic. All three of her daughters would become successful professional women.

As a young girl, I loved going to the movies. The Rialto Theatre was the one and only movie house in town, and little as it was, it became a fountain of dreams and aspirations. Through movies, I could escape to a glamorous life in faraway places, as far away from Alice, Texas, as my vivid imagination could take me. In my make-believe world I could live in Europe in a royal palace or a romantic villa where bad things never happened.

And so, when a lump appeared on Daddy's neck and was diagnosed as Hodgkin's disease, I wasn't grief-stricken or even surprised. It seemed to my teenage reasoning that eventually all that goes around really does come around. In fact, it was a kind of relief.

Mother brought us to his hospital room to discuss the situation. He lay there looking at us through an oxygen tent.

"Girls, Daddy and I need to talk to you." Mother had been crying.

"The doctors say he has just a few months to live. There is no cure. There is research going on in Houston on this kind of cancer. They want him there because it might help them find a cure for someone else, later. Or, he can spend his last months here with us. It's our decision. What do you girls want to do?"

It was a small room for such a big decision.

My sisters couldn't speak. Nor could Daddy. So I did.

"If he goes to Houston, at least some good could come of this, right? He's going to die anyway. Isn't it better to help someone instead of wasting away for nothing?"

It would prove to be a harsh sentence. Houston was 250 miles from home, meaning that his last months of life would be endured in a huge cancer ward without daily contact with family or friends. Most of the time he would be all alone.

Financially, we were devastated. Medical bills were mounting up, Mother was missing work without pay and, of course, we had no savings. We became a charity case for the church so that, for the four months Daddy was in Houston, we could drive up every week-end for regular visits. At times, we slept in the car, with only enough money for gas. Eventually, we were being summoned to Houston at any hour of the day or night.

"Come now. He may not make it through the night."

And, we would go.

It was Carmen's senior year in high school. I was a sophomore and Sylvia was in seventh grade.

A big, robust man whom we had feared as children was frail, emaciated by radiation treatments with bleeding gums and practically no hair. As we watched the changes in Daddy's appearance and in his character, a change came over us as well. We three sisters would walk huddled close together past rows and rows of beds occupied by men dying of cancer.

"Don't look at them." A whisper.

The ward was horrible and cold and smelled of death. Finally, we would come to the right bed and try to comfort this stranger who was occupying Daddy's body, or what was left of it. He now weighed seventy-five or eighty pounds.

Finally, there came a time when we knew it was the end. We were taking turns being with him so that he would not die alone. The bully who had lived his life as a coward, terrorizing his wife and daughters, was now a pitiful, little old man who would soon have to reconcile his life with God.

That last night it was my turn to relieve Mother and Sylvia, just before midnight. It was quiet on the ward except for the occasional hacking and coughing in the distance. Daddy opened his eyes and started to talk.

"Daddy, you should try and rest. Save your strength."

"I want you to know how sorry I am for everything. There's so much I've done wrong."

I looked at him with pity. Pity for him, afraid to die—and pity for us, a family scarred by years of damage.

And then he died. He was 44 years old.

That was my first experience with cancer. I was 15.

Today

It has been thirty-six years since those events of my childhood. During that time, I have had cancer twice; twice, I have recovered. What is different about the last episode is the profound way in which the experience changed me. My husband Rich and I fought the battle together, and together we won. More importantly, however, what we learned in the process of fighting it has radically altered the way I will spend the rest of my life. It changed my beliefs about faith and about God. This horrible illness that takes so many lives and shatters even more became a teacher for my family and me, and now we wish to share the benefits of our experience in the hope that they may be useful to others.

Three years have passed since the illness that threatened to take my life. I have virtually no lasting side effects from my treatments; I feel healthy and happy and have for many months. My life is in balance and my life choices are simpler. I have a broadened sense of humility and I know the meaning of love.

Of all that we learn about cancer, the most important lesson may be that we, as a society, learn to live with this disease until it can be cured. It is so prevalent in our lives that as a world community we must do a better job of assimilating it into our social structure. It has entered the mainstream and yet the acknowledgment of it is still closeted.

It was not until the year 2000 that the World Health Organization signed a charter outlining international standards of cancer treatment. This charter calls for eradicating stigmas surrounding the disease, improving access to clinical trials, better cancer screening, and greater emphasis on prevention initiatives. Already, more than five million people die from cancer every year worldwide. This number is predicted to double in the next twenty years.

These, however, are merely statistics. Cancer does not happen to human bodies; it happens to human beings. We are mothers and fathers, wives and husbands, sons and daughters, friends and lovers. When cancer strikes, everyone within the family circle becomes affected. The impact is always tremendous and sometimes catastrophic, yet it can also be a time of enormous spiritual and physical healing, a time of victory.

I have chosen to share my story in the hope that knowing one family's experiences may help others. This is a story about courage and faith and survival; of believing that, regardless of the statistics, miracles do occur. It is about taking control of life, even when it seems impossible to do so. Spiritually, it's of never giving up hope, and yet finding the strength to let go when your heart says it is time.

This is also a love story.

My husband and I have a deep, intense relationship that is based on the powerful love and great respect we have for each other. When we married five years before I became ill, we promised each other a lifetime of happiness, and we were living that promise. Then, suddenly, my illness threatened to change everything, threatened to break the vows we had made to live happily together into old age. Our world was suddenly and violently turned upside-down without a moment's notice, as is always the way with cancer.

It was during the very cold winter of 1998 when I became ill. The first chance we had to break away from our corporate jobs, Rich and I had escaped to Europe for a quick vacation right before

Christmas. On our last night in Paris, we walked for hours, finally arriving at an ice rink in the center of the city set against a backdrop of pure white trees sparkling with tiny crystal lights. And as we watched the skaters, enchanted as though in a dream, I distinctly remember thinking about how very far I'd come from Alice, Texas. I had a wonderful life.

The next day, excited to share a beautiful Christmas with the family, we returned to Oregon and suddenly our lives changed. We had been having so much fun . . . and then, it wasn't fun again for a very long time.

At the time, I could not have imagined the events that would engulf our lives in the following year. If I had been told what we would face, what we would learn and would do, I would have called it impossible. We did it. We did not choose to do it; we did it because we had to.

It is hard to believe that the journey that took us through the last few years could be so devastating and yet now seem so healed. Life is a series of decisions, and fortunately the decisions we would be forced to make with limited time and information would prove later to be right. Those decisions were never easy and there were many times when we were terrified that we might be wrong. Sometimes we reasoned correctly; sometimes we just got lucky.

We also believe in God, miracles, and prayer. Whether to restore the emotional and physical wellness, or to gather the needed strength to continue, we spoke to God and asked for His mercy. We were comforted when we felt lost. And ultimately, we were blessed with the strength to take responsibility for our situation. In the face of disaster we found the power to survive, the power to fight, and the power to heal.

Actually, I feel better than before my last battle with cancer. I am physically and emotionally strong and stable. More conscious of protecting the years ahead, I try to live my life more healthily.

Since my recovery, I cherish each new day differently. The small nuisances that distracted me before are now irrelevant, and the small treasures that seemed irrelevant before are now crystal clear.

These days, my life is extraordinarily happy and it is hard to imagine that it happened at all. It was a lifetime ago. My lifetime.

As I look back on our journey, it seems so far away, as though two other people we know and care about had gone through it, but not us. That is why the journey is presented here, with all its raw fear and joyful celebration, all the mistakes and the lessons—because the story must be told while I can still remember. My body's natural defense is working well. I am beginning to forget.

1

A Shocking Discovery

The day after Christmas, 1998 was one of those Oregon winter nights when the rain turns to sleet and the wind is bitter cold, the kind of night where you hate going out. So, even though it was my forty-ninth birthday, Rich and I decided to celebrate at home with my sister Sylvia, who was visiting from Texas. Later that night, Rich's son Scott and his wife Lynn arrived with a huge, decadent cake from a French bakery downtown, chocolate draped in chocolate with swirls and curls of chocolate on top. It was ridiculous and, of course, I couldn't resist it.

"Hey, you guys. This thing could kill me!"

Later that night I thought it would. A pain in my side began to build, and by two o'clock in the morning, I knew I was in real trouble.

"Honey, wake up. I think I need to go to the hospital."

I could feel a knife slicing through my side and into my back. I was having trouble breathing. This was not indigestion. Rich shook himself out of a deep slumber and dressed quickly, trying to grasp the seriousness of the situation. In fifteen minutes we were in the car and on our way to get help. It seemed like a very long ride.

Twenty minutes later, at the emergency room, I tried to describe my problem to the admitting nurse, then to the attending nurse, and then again to a doctor. I would explain the extreme level of pain two more times after that, wondering if anyone communicated in this chaotic environment and concluding that if they did, it was not on this shift. They were busy that night and holiday traffic had apparently brought in more serious cases than mine: a teenage boy thrown from a car, someone's grandmother who slipped on the ice, a baby bleeding and screaming, and more. The rooms were very full. So, even though Rich was demanding that I get attention, the best he could do was to commandeer a warm blanket as I lay in the cold examination room.

"Sir, emergency rooms are kept at lower temperatures to reduce the chances of infection," the nurse explained. "We'll be with you in a few minutes."

I lay there shivering from the cold, trying to be patient, my teeth now chattering because of the intensity of the pain. Finally, I was given something to "make you feel more comfortable."

I wasn't comfortable *at all*. I hated hospitals. I had been in emergency rooms before and there was nothing I could associate with comfort on that cold morning. Finally, as the clock approached 4:30, the narcotic kicked in.

With the pressure of the pain relieved, the cause of it was now the issue. X-rays were taken but they did not indicate any specific problem. They did, however, reveal that the lower part of my intestine was full and the attending doctor concluded that I had a partial bowel obstruction from prior surgeries.

"It happens sometimes when you heal from an old operation and scar tissue grows in the abdominal region," he said as he reviewed my medical history. "Let's see. You've had a tumor and gall bladder removed and a hysterectomy. That would create a fair amount of scar tissue in the area around the bowel. When the intestines pass food through the body, they move around, kind of like a snake. Sometimes these old scars get in the way and it causes them to kink up. We've given you a muscle relaxant and pain medication. Oh, and these laxatives."

It was that simple. I felt embarrassed for taking precious time and resources away from patients with real problems. It must have been that wicked cake after all.

And, so we went home, believing that everything was fine. The sun was starting to come up and the rain was yielding just a little bit. I would feel better after a long nap, and aided by the narcotic and being bone-tired, I slept most of the day.

When I awoke I didn't feel better at all. Once the drugs wore off, the pain recurred. It was insistent, throbbing, now more localized to my back. The laxatives had worked, so we ruled out the obstruction theory. I called my primary care physician, Dr. Van Sickle.

"It's in the wrong place for your appendix and you have no gall bladder. It's really hard to say what could be causing it. Why don't you go back to the hospital?"

I resisted. I did not want to go back. I wanted to be home with my husband. The thought of returning after hours of lying around in that cold room on a hard bed was abhorrent.

"Please don't make me go back. I spent hours there and they didn't find anything. Isn't there something we can do here? Maybe it's a pulled muscle. Maybe try a heating pad or a hot bath. It could just be sore from the kink in my gut," I offered a weak appeal, feeling guilty for bothering the doctor on his day off.

I should never have called. It's not really that bad.

"Dr. Van Sickle, I think I'm feeling a little better now than I was this morning . . . maybe we should see how I feel tomorrow." Now questioning my own judgment.

He must think I'm an idiot. I can't even describe the pain.

"Well, call me and let me know what's going on. If you start feeling better, fine. But let me know."

At midnight, I sat in a hot tub to numb the pain.

"Really, Rich, I think maybe it might be getting better." I was trying to convince myself as well as my husband. He wasn't buying it.

I slept awhile and then took another hot bath, over and over throughout the night. I popped Tylenol like M&Ms, but it wasn't going away. The next morning, I admitted defeat and called Dr. Van Sickle back.

"It's still there and it's getting worse. What do you think?" I asked, knowing what he would say, dreading what I would hear.

"Tell them I sent you back. Tell them I said to look for things in unlikely places. You've had so much prior surgery that it could be kind of confusing in there. Don't let them send you home until you are satisfied that we know exactly what's happening. That pain is there for a reason."

Indeed it was.

Now the pain intensified as though angry at my crude attempts to dismiss it. It was a deep, sharp stabbing and I thought that I would break in half from the force of it.

Rich drove me the twelve miles to the hospital, nervous now, rushing but trying not to be reckless as we passed dark streets in the freezing rain. I was moaning from the pain.

This is wrong. Very wrong.

As Rich hit the highway heading for the hospital, I crawled in torturous pain over the front seat of our SUV into the back, crying, rolling around, trying to crawl out of my own body. There was no relief.

"Hang on, baby, we're almost there."

Finally, back in the emergency room, we started all over again. Only this time I couldn't talk because the pain had escalated yet again.

"Please give her something for the pain, now." Rich tried anger, coercion, cornering anyone who came into my room. Again, what was normal procedure to the emergency room staff seemed to me to take an eternity. They were sympathetic and attentive and finally an hour after we arrived, a drug was infused into my veins and the pain became a dull ache.

"We're going to take a CT scan and see if we can solve this puzzle, Mr. Mattern. She'll be gone for a while. You may be more comfortable in the waiting room." A pleasant, efficient young doctor.

Rich held my hand until the last possible moment as they wheeled the gurney away.

An hour later, when the doctor returned with the test results, the look on his face was different from the open, relaxed smile he had an hour earlier. It was stressed, sobering. This was serious.

"Where is your husband?"

I knew that he would only ask me that if the news was bad, really bad.

"I think he went for coffee. Doctor, just tell me."

I had never shied away from a tough discussion; I braced myself for another.

"You have a mass on your pancreas. It's rather large. It seems to be pressing against the vein that runs along your spine. We think that's the source of the pain. We'd like to admit you to better understand your . . . options."

I knew from the look on his face that there would not be many. When Rich returned, I was shaking.

"It's the pancreas. He says I have a growth on the pancreas. They're admitting me," I said and began to cry. The implications of some rogue mass growing on my pancreas petrified me. The thoughts that flooded my mind, unwanted and unwelcome, pointed to one terrifying conclusion: I had cancer. Cancer of the pancreas.

I began feeling anxious, a slow but steady panic growing inside, making me frozen in fear. Rich bent down to hold me and I was enveloped in his tremendous warmth and incredible strength. It was he that kept me from going into shock, constantly reassuring me then and again in the days ahead. Whatever it was we would go through it together; together we would figure it out.

I was admitted immediately and began what would turn out to be many days of receiving increasingly bad news. There were numerous consultations, evaluations, and tests, mostly inconclusive. The vernacular changed. The "mass" was now being referred to as my "tumor," although we still did not know exactly what it was.

"The tumor is pushing against the superior vena cava, the major blood vessel to your heart. We think that's what's causing the pain." Dr. Swartz, my surgeon, explained.

Removal of the tumor seemed obvious to us, but evidently

there were serious surgical concerns.

"Before we decide to go in, I'd like as much information about this thing as I can get. A lot of things can happen in surgery. The more we can prepare for it, the more predictable the outcome will be. It's in a very tricky place."

Dr. Swartz was being very cautious; we would only get one shot at this.

One procedure to examine the chemistry of the tumor involved insertion of a device with tiny claws through a small incision in the abdomen. The claws were designed to pinch off pieces of tissue so that biopsies could be conducted. I imagined an arcade game for picking up toy prizes that seem to be easily reachable but are not. The three attempts to extract tissue were unsuccessful. The biological properties of the growth were still unknown, so there was no way to decide exactly what to do.

Across the country, friends and colleagues returning to work after New Year's were just getting the news of my condition. Rich and I waited, frustrated and frightened, while flowers from friends and business associates began to fill my hospital room.

2

The Surgery

At this point, although our most pressing problem was removal of the tumor, I sensed a hesitation or discomfort from Dr. Swartz.

"The surgery is called a Whipple procedure. What we plan to do is go in through the abdominal wall, remove the tumor and any areas that may be involved with it, and assuming all goes as planned, connect everything back up again."

"So, what are the risks?" I wanted to know everything.

"Well, we have several risks. First, this tumor could be getting its blood from the vein it's pressing against. We just can't tell from the X-rays or any other tests we've been running. If it is, removal of the tumor would be like cutting directly into that major vein and we wouldn't be able to stop the blood flow."

"You're saying I would bleed to death?"

"Yes."

I understood all of the words he was using but was working hard to comprehend their meaning. It may have been the morphine coursing through my veins to stem the pain; it may have been my disbelief that we were negotiating death, my death.

"Do I have any other options?"

"If we leave the tumor in, there are several possible consequences. It could rupture and again, if the vena cava is the blood source, the hemorrhaging will be fatal. Or, it may not be feeding directly from the vena cava, but could still be cancerous. In that case, cancer cells could infiltrate the bloodstream and metastasize, spreading cancer throughout the body. Remember, this tumor is still growing and we can't stop your pain unless we do something about the tumor. On the other hand, if you don't want to risk the surgery, we can try to make you comfortable until the tumor takes over."

He was talking about going home to die. Masking the pain and going away to die. As he said it I became strangely detached from the conversation. I began to wonder what it was like for him, carefully selecting every word, practiced and deliberate. I wondered if he wished he could comfort us and reassure us with his competence, his years of training, and his command of modern medicine. I was strangely sympathetic, as though I were watching a soap opera and in this episode the young, handsome doctor has a bad day; he has to break the news.

We had only two choices: a high-risk surgery that I might not survive or dying slowly in a few weeks or months from the tumor. It was incomprehensible that these were my choices. I was still in a state of disbelief that this could be happening. Then, the colossal implications of the prognosis began to sink in, not crashing—sudden and loud—but crushing, as though the sky became heavy and began pushing against the earth. The odds were in favor of my dying. I would probably die. I became lost in sorrow.

We needed privacy. Rich asked the nurses to stop all procedures; everything could wait. Please, please, no visitors. No calls. No lab technicians. Nothing. No one. Please. We needed to be alone.

Rich stayed by my side, afraid even to step out to talk to the nurses, afraid that I might suddenly break the last thread keeping me from drowning in my own fear. Steadfastly refusing to give up hope, he spoke to me over and again of his optimism, his genuine belief in his heart of hearts that I would be well again.

"We're not done yet, you and me. We have so much to do together."

Rich took me to the chapel and together we prayed for clarity of thought to make the right decision and for the strength to live with the consequences.

A few hours later, Dr. Van Sickle came to see me. He had been tracking my case since I was admitted and had been in consultation with the surgeon, sharing his concern about the position of the tumor.

"I'm worried that he's worried," I told him.

"Well, this is not a simple operation. A Whipple's actually just about as complicated as surgery gets. It will involve removing part of the pancreas and possibly some other organs. It all depends on what Dr. Swartz discovers when he goes in. There could be other troublesome spots that worry him once he gets a better look. And then, of course, he has to reconnect all those parts, your organs and valves, and try to get them working again."

This sounded very ambitious.

"Will it work? I mean, assuming I survive the operation, will all those things reconnect just like that, like so much plumbing?"

"Theoretically it should work. The gastro-intestinal system is just that—a system. Digestion is an elaborate process. It requires movement of food through different parts of the body that convert it into nutrients that are absorbed into the bloodstream and used by the body. The Whipple isn't our biggest problem right now. If it doesn't work, we have alternative methods for feeding the body.

"Removing the tumor is our main concern. Now, if all goes as planned, Dr. Swartz will go in and extract it, then we'll conduct biopsies and then—well, then we'll know what we're up against."

I was fascinated with how precise the doctors were with their choice of words and how they were being very careful not to give me false hopes. However, Dr. Van Sickle was someone we knew and trusted; I knew I was getting it straight. If there were more to know, we would know it.

I also knew Dr. Swartz, although not as well. He had removed my gall bladder two years earlier. This, however, was clearly not a gall bladder operation. It was major-league surgery. How good was he?

"Kim Swartz is a fine, fine technician. He knows what to do and how to do it as well as any surgeon. I'm very confident with him. I think you can be too."

The only real potential option for survival was the surgery. So, although the risks were very high, we decided to go ahead. I would be going into surgery with the odds of returning against me.

Rich had not been spending the night at the hospital. Every day he would stay until I was able to sleep and then go home for the night and return the next morning. The morning of my surgery, a miscommunication of the operating room schedule meant I was going into surgery an hour earlier than we expected.

"But . . . but my husband's not here yet."

"I'm sorry, but we have to go now. Everything's ready and the doctors are waiting."

I panicked. I tried calling Rich but couldn't get through. What if I didn't survive? What would he do? How would he feel about not saying goodbye because he had to stop at the cleaners or the bank? It would be awful not to have said, "I love you."

Quickly, I wrote him a note telling him my last thoughts of him . . . of us. I left it on my bed, realizing that he would come in and not find me.

Oh Rich, My Darling Rich —
I wanted them to wait just long
enough for you to come. But no!
I couldn't do it. We had to go!
So this is not Good Bye.

Please know that I am calm, at peace thinking of you. That every thought as I go down will be of you – of us. Happy thoughts as you have made me so.

I'll close my eyes to see your face, to take you with me when I go.

You came into my life and changed my very being. You touched my body and my spirit and made me yours forever.

I love you.

I love you.

Annette

And then I prayed.

In addition to the morphine, I had been given something to make me relax for the surgery. I tried to clear my mind and talk to God. I prayed for myself and for Rich and for our family. The edges of my mind became hazy, as though I were in a dream. I was having trouble staying focused. I prayed for Rich to come, as much for him as for myself.

They transferred me to a gurney, preparing me to go. Voices. I heard voices in the distance, a kind of echoing sound. I struggled to understand.

"We're going to move you now. Are you okay?" The orderly in green scrubs was moving things around me, tubes and cords, tying me to poles like some giant, grotesque marionette.

"Are you okay?'

"Yes, I think so." I tried to slow my breathing.

God, give me strength. I tried not to be scared.

"I'm going to put you in the hall a minute. Then we'll be going downstairs, okay?"

The buzz of another day, a day just like every other day on the fourth floor of St. Vincent's Hospital, seemed so normal to everyone else. But I was not okay.

Rich, where are you? Please, God, please take care of him ... and ... and ...

Tears.

"Ma'am, are you okay?"

No, I was not okay. Maybe we had made a mistake. Maybe I shouldn't have the surgery. After all, the odds weren't that great. Maybe I should just cherish the next few days or weeks or months or whatever God would give me. Maybe that was my time to be with Rich, to say goodbye to the people I love. Maybe they could just medicate me and send me home. No, I was not okay.

Oh, dear God, please help me.

I tried to remember the prayers of my childhood. The realization that this could be the last conversation, the last touch, the last sight I might have emerged like a demon from the dark corners of my mind.

"What's going on?"

I heard his voice like a distant memory, unsure if it was the drug or my imagination.

"Annette, what's going on?"

His voice clearer now, punctuated by the urgency of his footsteps. I lifted my head but couldn't see very well. I was afraid to believe in the little miracle.

"Rich?" My voice seemed tiny, as though a part of me were already gone.

The orderly came out of my room with my medical chart and put it on the blanket that covered my feet.

"Rich, are you here?" I didn't let myself believe until he touched me. Yes, he was real and he was here. I was not alone. A single prayer had been heard and had been answered. He leaned over the gurney and held me and kissed me as we started to move toward the elevators.

"Sir, you can go downstairs with us. There's a waiting room where we'll come and get you when she's done."

"Annette, what's going on? I thought . . ." Rich balanced his confusion with his instinct to protect and support me.

The hall was long and narrow. We passed door after door and the name on each one was a blur. We seemed to be entering a chamber.

"I . . . tried . . . to call you. I . . . I couldn't . . ." I looked for words that had just been there.

"I am so, so sorry. Oh, honey, I didn't want to wake you too early. I was on the phone with your mother and then stopped to get chains on the car. They think it might snow." Snow? I had been encapsulated in my environmentally controlled cocoon for so long that I had lost my sense of the outside world. Of course, he would leave late tonight; he would be tired and it would be dark. Of course.

"All that matters is you're here now. I love you."

"I love you too, baby. You're going to be fine. I know you're going to be fine. Are you okay?"

Yes, now I was okay.

I have no memory of the surgery after that.

3

$\mathcal{R}$*ich*

On April 16, 1945, Rich Mattern was born in Aberdeen, South Dakota, and adopted at birth. Red hair and freckles and all, he would be taken home and loved and spoiled by his new parents who had longed for a child until well into their forties. His world would be perfect for a little boy with toys and clothes and a big, black dog. Then, at the age of three, his adoptive mother would succumb to cancer of the liver. His father, heartbroken and miserable, would move to Portland near his sister Marion, who could help with his son. A fire captain in Aberdeen, the widower found work in Oregon on a farm. And it was there, one day when Rich was seven, that the boy would discover his dad dead from a heart attack. The scream would alert neighbors a mile away.

Aunt Marion and her husband took the boy in, even though their modest home in a blue-collar neighborhood was already full with three children of their own. So, a six-by-eight-foot room without heat would be carved out of the garage, and there, Richie Mattern would live until he went to college.

He would marry, father three children: Tracy, Scott, and Kelly, and settle in Lake Oswego, a suburb of Portland. His first priority would be his family, and he reared his children to be loving, caring people. In time, as the children started their own families, he would become "Papa Richie" to the grandchildren who would happily enter his world.

His marriage didn't last, although his zest for life did. Over the years Rich would be known for his sense of humor and his exuberant personality. He would have friends for a lifetime; little boys who played together at eight or nine years old were still close friends forty years later. Ambitious and hard working, he developed a keen sense of business and eventually became an executive of DuPont.

And then we met.

It was a blind date. It started out as a casual dinner. Then, his charm wrapped itself around me like a velvet cape and I fell in love. Over the next six months we discovered that we shared the same values and dreams and aspirations. It was New Year's Eve, as we kissed at midnight on the dance floor, that he proposed.

"I want to spend every New Year with you for the rest of my life."

It was perfect. This is the man I was supposed to meet, to know and love and be loved by. We brought meaning to each other; our laughter was deeper, with greater understanding because we were together. On a beautiful autumn day, we married, honeymooned in Europe, and began living a dream come true.

Now, Rich sat in the waiting room. Two of his friends who had been buddies since childhood came to keep vigil with their friend. They understood the gravity of the situation and would be sure that Rich was not alone. They recounted stories they had told a million times of school days and college days and just the other day. It didn't matter; the banter was sufficiently distracting from the stress of uncertainty.

The hours passed; the morning was gone.

Then, to Rich's surprise, my sister Sylvia appeared in the doorway of the waiting room. She had been with us for Christmas and had returned to Texas the day I was first sent home from the hospital. A schoolteacher with four teenage children still living at home with her and her husband, she nevertheless had managed the quick turnaround for my surgery.

Rich couldn't understand how she could be here, standing in the waiting room, dragging her luggage behind her.

"I got off the plane, found a bus to the light rail, went downtown, switched to another bus, transferred one more time, and ended up here. Did you know there's a bus that drops you off right here in front of the hospital?"

They were speechless. She had found her way to the suburban hospital twenty miles from the Portland airport. She knew she had to be here.

Sylvia joined Rich and his two friends for a long wait. The surgery lasted eight hours.

Editor's Note:
This is the first of a series of drawings taken from the author's jour-
nal. You will find others strategically placed in accordance with the
time line of her experiences. Through them you will be able to more
clearly relate to her mindset of the moment.

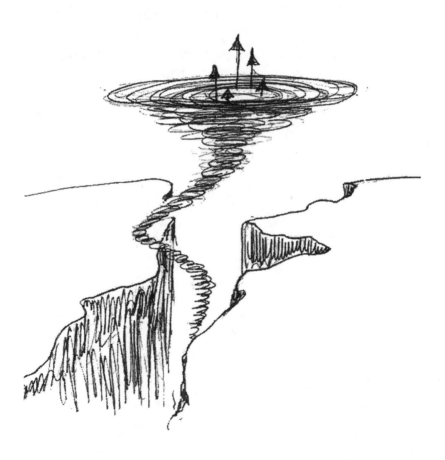

You are a force - like a whirlwind -
that sucks me out of the abyss
of the ordinary.

4

Harsh Consciousness

I heard a man's voice softly yelling at me through a fog.

"Can you hear me?"

There was an echo in the sound.

"I need for you to wake up. I'm going to move you around. Can you hear me?"

I thought I was strapped down to a table with restraints on my arms and legs. The table was moving in all directions at once, like a gyroscope. It was making me dizzy.

"I want you to move now. We need to move, okay?"

Move? Couldn't he see that was impossible? What was wrong with him? I was strapped down, my arms and legs restrained and completely immobile. Besides, the table was spinning and surely I would fall off.

"You're all done, ma'am. You're in recovery now and we need to move. It's real important that we move. We're going to do it together. Do you understand?"

My vision came into focus. Yes, I would help him move. In a single moment the realization came over me that I was alive, here in a recovery room, and I now needed to cooperate with the people who had saved my life. Whatever it took, I had to move.

"Yes... okay." I said, or perhaps I thought; I really don't know which.

My next awareness was the physical awakening of my shattered body, as though I had been a rag doll torn apart by an angry dog, then sewn back together, her stuffing not quite like before.

It wasn't a table after all. It was a bed and it did move. I knew it! It was lifting at my head slowly 15 degrees, then 30, and then 45. I envisioned myself a pile of dirt on the bed of a dump truck that was lifting at one end and, at any minute, I might tumble onto the floor. But the recovery room nurse was a strong young man and he held me firmly in place. He took my limbs and then my torso and made me do what his training had taught him was necessary for my successful recovery. I felt barely alive. My muscles and tissues and nerves were screaming.

"Pa...pain." I licked my lips trying to talk, my mouth dusty dry.

"Okay, just stay with me. You're doing fine. We'll get you something for the pain. I just need you to wake up for me."

I drifted in and out.

"Annette?" I was dreaming about Rich and my sister.

"Annette? Honey, how are you doing? Annette?"

I opened my eyes and Rich stood over me.

"Sylvia's here," he said, still amazed that she was with us, sharing the surprise with me.

"I know." I don't know how I knew, but I did know. And I drifted back to sleep.

The next day the full implications of the surgery would become apparent. The tumor was sent to pathology and the mechanical process of recovery from an impossible surgery began.

"We removed the head of the pancreas, which was nearly engulfed by the tumor. Fortunately, it was not feeding directly from the vena cava so we removed it without too much complication. We also removed about half of your stomach, the duodenum, and sections of the bowel. Basically, we had to extract everything that was in contact with the tumor because of contamination. We also did a very thorough visual examination, however, and we couldn't see any other growths that looked abnormal."

Dr. Swartz had been the right choice after all.

"You've just undergone extensive surgery and what we need right now is for you to heal. Your vital signs are good and I'm optimistic about your recovery. The next order of business is to get your digestive system working again. In the meantime, we'll let you know when we get results back from pathology on the outcome of the biopsy. For now, just focus on getting better from the surgery."

I had tubes jutting out of my neck, a simple bandage securing a shunt to my jugular, like a water spigot on the neck of a cartoon character. Now three intravenous bags replaced the one I had before and, besides the catheter, I had machines everywhere. As I closed my eyes and carefully touched the drainage bulbs protruding from my abdomen, I wondered how I would live from now on, for I had never imagined myself here.

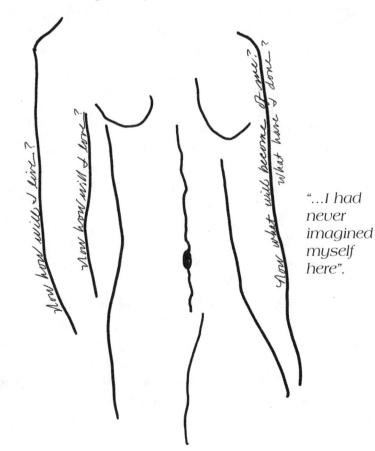

"...I had never imagined myself here".

For several years, one of Sylvia's children had been treated for a rare gastro-intestinal condition at the best hospitals in the country, from UCLA to the Mayo Clinic. Her knowledge of and familiarity with medical procedures and systems was encyclopedic for a layperson. Now, from morning until bedtime, she stayed by my side questioning every procedure, every medication. She asked the nurses to explain each monitor so that we knew what was being watched and why. Often the staff used "med-speak" and she would translate for me into common language. And she ensured that each nurse and technician who entered my room first washed his or her hands or put on new gloves before working on me.

"They get in a hurry and just forget. Or, they get called out and when they come back in, they could be contaminated. Remember, everybody here is sick. Hospitals are loaded with germs. We have to be very diligent about trying to maintain a germ-free environment to the extent that we can. You have an incision here that is extremely susceptible to infection."

One day she arrived with a spiral notebook that I assumed was something she was working on for her class. The class, as it turned out, was to be here in my room.

"We need to start writing everything down," she said. "When I first started interacting with the doctors and nurses, I was absolutely positive that I could remember everything they were telling me, but I was wrong. Sometimes I would have a different recollection than others who had heard the same conversation. Or, I would confuse a discussion I'd had with one doctor with that of another. So, I started making notes, something I could refer to later with names and dates and what each discussion was about.

"Remember, this is all new to you and while you're still trying to process what they just said, they're giving you more information. Plus, you have no frame of reference. If you don't keep some kind of record it gets very convoluted—especially for someone on pain meds."

Sylvia began teaching me about the world of long-term medical care, lessons about understanding procedures and challenging decisions in a positive, productive way.

"The best advice I can give you is not to accept anything you don't fully comprehend. If it isn't clear, ask again or get them to write it down. Don't be uncomfortable about insisting on a clear explanation. You have a right to know everything that's being done to you. It's your responsibility to yourself, to Rich, and the rest of us, even to the doctors."

Every day she got me up to walk, all the while imparting her vast knowledge of hospital routines and procedures.

"I think the most frustrating thing is some medical people just don't listen to their patients. They make assumptions based on experience or training, and generally they're right. But, we nearly lost a child because one doctor dismissed my cautions about his unique condition. You must be your own advocate."

Up and down the halls we would go, dragging my pumps and infusions with us, walking to ignite the paralyzed nerves of my bowel while waiting for news of the tumor. Rich's daughter Tracy began making daily visits to the hospital to be sure there was always someone with us.

For several days the family waited for news from the lab. In my hospital room, flowers continued to arrive like new recruits relieving the tired soldiers whose mission was to mask the sterile environment in which I now lived. The waiting seemed interminable.

When I was first admitted, a resident doctor who was on the periphery of my case had made a small but careless mistake. We had called him on it and since then he had sought to reassure us of his competence. As the resident, he was our normal access to information about what was happening with my case. Every day on his rounds, it was the same conversation.

"Any news yet, Doctor?"

"No. Nothing."

Finally, one day, he came excitedly into my room and proceeded to announce the results of the biopsy.

"Good news!" He announced it with a big smile from ear to ear. "It's benign. There's no evidence of cancer."

We thanked God and we rejoiced and called our friends and

family. We laughed and cried. Then, Sylvia, with new lightness in her heart, went home to her family.

The next day, Dr. Swartz came to examine me and to talk.

"The biopsy is back and the tumor is malignant. I'm sorry but it's definitely cancer."

It was shocking, utterly unbelievable.

You're wrong. The other doctor told us . . .

"It seems to have initiated with the pancreas. However, that's not my area of specialty. Oncologists, cancer specialists, are the ones who determine treatment options once they examine the pathology report. That will take a couple of days. There is a Tumor Board that convenes on Tuesdays. It's there that the pathologists and other specialists will get together to discuss your case. They are the ones who make recommendations on treatment and they'll be able to give you an idea of what's next. I'm sorry that we don't have better news."

I felt as if I had been slapped and could feel the heat of my face and the sting of my skin. Rich and I were both stunned. We knew, of course, that Dr. Swartz was right. The other doctor had made another mistake. In his zeal to tell us good news, he set us up for a bigger fall.

The realization that what I had in fact was cancer had the effect of a powerful, dark force gripping me at the throat and pulling me off the cliff of fear. I was falling, down . . . down . . . down . . .

"Annette, listen to me." Rich's voice was insistent and he was looking straight into my face as I brought him into focus.

"Let's not worry about that now," pulling me back. "We don't really know what we're dealing with yet. That is just one piece of information. We don't know enough to be scared. Right now, let's just work on healing from the surgery. That's all we're supposed to be doing right now, remember?"

Once I was settled, Rich left to talk to the head of the hospital, still furious that I had been given false hope. He told them that the resident doctor with the misdiagnosis was never to come to my room again. I was no longer his patient.

At this point, although we knew it was cancer, we were not being told definitively what kind or whether the prognosis was good or bad. It would be several days before the conclusions of the Tumor Board would be known. Another very long wait.

Rich's great love for his children was mirrored in his daughter Tracy's sensitivity to the situation. Beyond her concern for me, she could feel her father's fear and pain and decided that she would experience it with him. As a distraction for me from the stress of waiting, she often brought along on her six-year-old son, Chris, and Jonny, his three-year-old brother.

"Hi, Gramma Net."

"Hi, Gramma Net."

"Hi, boys."

They were fascinated by the menagerie of machines and tubes and gadgets that seemed to be growing out of me.

"Gramma Net, we made you some art work for your room," Chris, the spokesman, said. "Here, Gramma."

"Here, Gramma," echoed Jonny.

And I would look at these two beautiful children and wonder if I would be here as they grew up. Would I know Chris's best teacher or Jonny's favorite sport? Would I see them learn to dance and go to prom? Drive a car? Go to college? Fall in love? Would they remember me? They were so young.

But, Tracy knew. She knew with wisdom beyond her years that they would leave me with more than artwork on my hospital room wall. They would leave me with a longing for more time, time to be a grandmother to children of the children I didn't have. She had brought the greatest gift of all: the immortality that comes of loving and teaching another generation.

"Bye, Gramma Net."

"Bye, Gramma Net."

"Bye, boys."

5

Cancer

Many types of cancer are known to exist; some are treatable, some not. And their treatments vary, based on the specific type of cancer, the stage of the illness, and the overall condition of the patient. Before decisions can be made about possible therapies or other courses of action, the cancer must be classified. The broad categories of the disease include cancers of the bone, brain, breast, endocrine system, lungs, skin, bladder, and kidney. There are cancers of the head and neck, leukemia, lymphomas, myelomas, sarcomas, and gastrointestinal cancers, including colorectal and pancreatic cancer. Some cancers affect only men, such as genitourinary cancer. The gynecologic cancers, such as ovarian, cervical, endometrial, and vulvar cancers, affect only women. Some cancers affect only adults; some, only children.

Cancerous tumors are further defined by comparing their microscopic features to those of healthy tissues, measuring the degree of abnormality versus normal cells. This process, called "Grade," categorizes most tumors by four degrees of severity, beginning with Grade 1 for low-grade tumors through Grades 3 and 4 for the most aggressive tumors. Some cancers use different grading systems to more appropriately define the various differences in the clinical behavior of the disease, as with prostate cancer.

Further classification, called "Stage," describes the extent to which the cancer has progressed and is particularly concerned with whether or not the disease has spread to other parts of the body. These factors, combined with the general condition of the patient, impact the distinct treatment plan for each individual.

In my case, the location of the tumor on the pancreas was a fairly strong indication that I had pancreatic cancer. This diagnosis would have been devastating. According to the American Cancer Society, eighty percent of the cases of pancreatic cancer are diagnosed so late that no effective treatment exists for them. Mine was a large, mature tumor, sure to draw a death sentence. The facts gave us little reason for optimism.

My doctors, however, were dogged in pursuit of better options. Although I had responded to numerous questionnaires about my medical history and had listed prior surgeries related to cancer, my current problem was being approached as an unrelated illness. However, once a connection was made with my gynecologist, Dr. Oscar Polo, the course was changed. He explained when he came to see me.

"I told them that twelve years ago you had a rare form of ovarian cancer called granulosa cell. I believed it was possible for this to be a recurrence. I had your records from Virginia, but we needed slides of the actual cancer cells to be sure. The problem was that it was so long ago that it was unlikely that the hospital would still have them. Usually they dispose of these records after eight or nine years."

I was confused about how this could be ovarian cancer if it was on the pancreas.

"We classify cancer by type when and where it first occurs—in your case, the ovaries or ovarian cancer. A recurrence of cancer means the cancer cells were not thoroughly eradicated with the previous treatment and the cells moved through the body, reseeding in another location. I believed your old cancer had simply found a suitable host, your pancreas, and was silently growing there all this time."

Growing there all this time?

Each word fell on me like a boulder, smashing my beliefs about my body for the last twelve years. Like some demon spawn, a cancerous tumor had grown from my cells. I could imagine it feeding on me, nurtured by me, and yet its purpose was to kill me. I forced myself to return to his conversation.

"We needed more information before we knew for sure. Some cancers look and act similarly although their reaction to treatment would be radically different. Also, there was little agreement about your case . . . which is good. That's the purpose of the Tumor Board—to give the experts a forum to review all the facts we have available and to debate the possible options. We look at every point of view and then reach a decision about what we're dealing with and what to do about it. We believe that, in that way, we come up with the best approach to treating each individual patient. Although we learn a lot about cancer from patterns, we must look at each case as unique. That's why it was critical in your case that we get as much information as we could about your previous condition.

"So, we contacted Arlington Hospital, even though it was a long shot. If at all possible, we felt that it was essential that we compare their records to the new pathology report. It took quite a long time to get confirmation but . . . what do you know? There they were. By some miracle, Arlington had detailed slides of your original tumor. It was a perfect match." Dr. Polo's smile spread across his face, pleased with the outcome.

I should have been pleased as well, knowing that pancreatic cancer was ruled out. This was incredibly good news, but somehow, the emotional shock of what was happening to me was overwhelming my ability to reason through it. I was angry that I had been unknowingly carrying around this illness for years, feeling ignorant of my own body. And, I could not understand how I could be dying now, now that I had attained what I had worked all my life to achieve.

My life with Rich had become an immeasurable source of love, support, and fun. We both worked hard and enjoyed professional success in the corporate world. We were active with our family and in our community. I had a very good life and was incredibly happy. This just couldn't be happening. Not to me. Not now. I had already battled this insidious disease. And I had already won once.

6

The First Occurrence

In 1983 my former husband and I were living in the Bay Area of California. Once my two stepdaughters, Teri and Cindy, were out of school and on their own, I had time to focus on advancing my career, which I did, accepting a promotion with AT&T to the federal government headquarters for the company in Washington D.C., where I had lived previously in the mid 1970s.

There were many positive aspects to moving back to Washington. My new business responsibilities created a solid foundation for my future career; working at the epicenter of world politics was tremendously exciting; and the relationships I developed helped me to grow personally and professionally. In addition, I formed a significant friendship with a woman who would become my new best friend, Shirley.

Shirley and I could not have been more different. She was a born Washingtonian who had lived in the nation's capital all her life. She epitomized understated elegance, was smart and preppy, with an insider's knack for east-coast style, sharp and chic. We worked in the same office, contracting telecommunications and computer systems to the Department of Defense. From the very beginning there was perfect communication between us; she knew exactly what I meant and I knew the same of her. We found that we also had in common a sense of humor that was rampant and unbridled, and we quickly became pals. Shirley and I worked best as a team, first at AT&T, then again several years later when we moved to USWEST.

For the seven years we worked together, our time was creative, interesting, and challenging because we approached the work that way. We also honed our skills at working with heads of government and dealing within bureaucratic structures, experiences that taught me a great deal about political and organizational dynamics. I gained from Shirley a more polished style and decorum that would aid me greatly in my career. She says she learned from me the importance of being natural in the business world, making an asset of "being herself."

I was always impressed with Shirley's ability to open any door in the most important city in the world. She understands the maze and navigates it adroitly—knows the secret handshake. Once, we were invited to lunch with a friend of hers at his private club downtown. As we arrived at the elegant Federal-style residence discreetly located near George Washington University, the doorman addressed us by name as though we were regular guests. We, of course, had never been there before. We entered reverently and my eyes took in rooms appointed in the very finest examples of American antiques, furnishings of museum quality. Having grown up in this environment, Shirley found this perfectly normal.

"The club is so private that for years the names of the members were not written down at all," our host was almost whispering. "Now, there is only one membership log which is handwritten and is kept by the dowagers."

"So tell me, does the President ever dine here?" I asked, fascinated.

"Not unless a member invites him."

It was part of the Washington ladder that commoners never see, way up at the top. Shirley didn't live in those circles but she could operate there with finesse. Whether it was a Presidential inauguration or a top brass affair, Shirley could get us there.

In 1987 that expertise made Shirley essential to a project we took on at the request of a good friend and colleague, Tom, a director from our manufacturing division. Our goal was to spotlight a strategic new product that could elevate our position in the competitive world of government technology. As co-chairs, Tom and I spent weeks devising maps and diagrams to steer the gigantic AT&T machine and its valuable resources. Confident with our plans, we launched a major publicity campaign, crowing about capabilities the development team had promised us. Then, things started to go wrong.

Systems were failing and critical functions were missing, with no indication of progress. Short delays turned into weeks and weeks turned into months—months we did not have to spare. While Tom and I wrestled with factory setbacks and logistical hurdles, we watched our project plunge into deep jeopardy. Finally, we reached our "drop dead" date, the last possible opportunity for turning back. After agonizing over it, Tom and I eventually committed ourselves to the impossible: we would complete the project.

Tom's conference room became a war room staffed with people commandeered from other jobs. They threw out the beautiful multicolored charts, then "short-cut" through each department. We juggled scores of calendars for the product launch, from the media to the Washington elite, buying time with the key guests whose attendance was the measure of our success. Nothing less than a flawless execution would be acceptable. For the few remaining weeks, we worked virtually nonstop, managing the pieces hands-on. Shortly before the event, the last hurdle fell; all the pieces fit. Finally able to relax a bit, Tom and I decided to take the weekend off so that we would be fresh for the senior management briefing the following Monday.

My weekend, however, was not restful. I felt horrible. My husband and I argued the entire time about my long work hours. Meanwhile, I ignored the ache in my abdomen by consuming whatever I could find to mask the pain. By Monday, what I assumed was menstrual cramps aggravated by extreme fatigue became so severe that I could hardly walk.

My timing could not have been worse. On the very day that could make or break my career, I could not get out of bed. At the last possible moment, I gave in and called Tom.

"I don't think I should drive," I said, sounding incoherent even to myself. "I'm not feeling . . . well . . . had a terrible . . . I don't suppose you can hold off until tomorrow?"

I remember feeling weak and dizzy as I tried to explain, my breathing deliberate and labored. If only I could close my eyes and sleep.

"Annette, I don't like the sound of this."

"Tom. I'm fine. Look, I'll bounce back . . . I just can't seem to . . . right now."

"Listen, I think you need some help. Now, hang up the phone and call 911." His voice was adamant. "911, Annette."

"Don't be silly." My voice now a whisper even to myself. "If I could just . . . a nap . . . a short nap."

"Annette." The alarm in his voice clashed with his typical laid-back drawl. "Listen, now. Listen to me. Are you doin' it or am I? 'Cause one of us is calling 911—now."

By the time I arrived at the hospital, my pain had somehow faded without medication and I was drifting away on a summer breeze, strangely calm while everyone around me seemed agitated, rushing around with monitors and needles. They talked about me although I didn't seem to be part of it at all.

"Her veins have collapsed."

Everyone rushed around me, tense and nervous, ordering things about. In contrast, I felt peaceful, rested, and strangely unafraid.

"Get Pediatrics down here and see if they can get—"

"Get that nail polish off."

But I have an important meeting, said the voice in my head.

The nurse with the polish remover looked silly running beside the gurney as I was being whisked down the hall, chattering on about their needing to see changes in the color of the nail.

"What's wrong with me?"

A doctor came in and everyone seemed to talk at once, but I

couldn't hear because of a ringing in my ears.

"What's wrong with me, Doctor?"

"We don't know, exactly. But it is serious and I think we need to get in there now to see what's going on inside. Instead of waiting for tests or X-rays, we're going to just go in there now so we can figure it out. I want you to start counting backwards . . ."

When the doctor visited me in recovery, I learned how very lucky I was. He explained that a grapefruit-size tumor had grown around my right ovary and had ruptured, causing internal hemorrhaging for two or three days. In the process, I had spilled half of my blood supply into my abdominal cavity, thus marinating my internal organs in roughly five liters of blood and triggering their eventual breakdown. Too much blood, he said. So much that "our only concern was to stop you from dying."

The operation required irrigation and repositioning of nearly every organ in the abdominal area, after removal of the tumor and its ovarian host. Although visual examinations of the remaining tissue revealed nothing unusual to the naked eye, as a matter of routine, the doctor ordered a biopsy.

"Are you talking about cancer?" I knew it, and yet I couldn't believe it.

"The only way to determine for certain is to examine it in the pathology lab. Many ovarian tumors are benign. It's not always cancer. Let's just wait and see."

We did, and it was.

"It's called granulosa cell. It's a fairly rare type of ovarian cancer. The group it's in, the stromal tumors, represents only five percent of cancers as a total group and granulosa cell is a subset of that. We don't see it very often but we do know this: it is definitely malignant."

The doctor had to say it several times before it sunk in.

"Malignant."

My knowledge of cancer in women was limited to breast cancer and that was what I had feared all of my adult life. Not ovarian cancer. In fact, I knew very little about ovarian cancer.

"Ovarian cancers are a very nasty group. You see, they don't give us warning signs until it's very late. We don't know why you got it because we don't know what causes it."

Was I going to die?

Not today, he said. Not today.

"However, you have a decision to make. We left the rest of your reproductive tissue in place, including the remaining ovary. Judging by the size of this tumor, it had been in there awhile, with ample opportunity to shed cells to nearby tissue. Also, when you hemorrhaged, cancerous cells could have spread through the blood."

I was stunned.

"My recommendation is to go home for a month and give your body a rest. Then, a month from now, we'd like you back for another operation. A hysterectomy. I believe we need to take out the rest of your reproductive organs and tissues. It would be a radical hysterectomy; everything goes. It's the only way to be sure the cancer won't spread."

Cancer. And a hysterectomy. All at once.

"Is that my only option? What about chemotherapy?"

"Chemotherapy hasn't been effective with this cancer. The only way to contain the disease is to cut it out. We need to remove any breeding ground where the cells could attach and nest. Otherwise, it will probably come back and it will eventually kill you."

The second operation would reveal the same cancer, granulosa cell, growing on the remaining ovary. So, the decision to remove my reproductive system at age thirty-seven proved to be right: the cancer had spread.

For the preceding two years, I had experienced excessive bleeding and cramping but had put it out of my mind. I was conditioned to ignore the pain.

"You can't spend a week in bed every month of your life," Mother would reprimand us growing up. Not wanting us to be weak, she would regale us with the wisdom of the non-slacker. "Housework is the best cure for cramps," she would say. It had been a family joke for years.

I had let those last two years go by without listening to my body, blind to the small signs of danger. My calendar was too busy to schedule a checkup and my Pap test was long overdue. However, because I hadn't liked my gynecologist, I hadn't been conscientious about my examinations. Well, now I had a new doctor, a cancer specialist.

Later I would learn that ovarian cancer ranks fifth as the cause of cancer deaths and is the sixth most common cancer in women. The American Cancer Society estimated that in the year 2000 there were about 23,100 new cases of ovarian cancer in this country and about fourteen thousand women who died of the disease. Ovarian cancer causes more deaths than any other reproductive organ disease. Many women believe that regular Pap tests are a sufficient monitor for all gynecologic cancers, and they ignore other warning signs being sent by their bodies. Many of us are embarrassed to complain, stigmatized about our "female problems." Unfortunately, ovarian cancer does not show up on Pap tests and early detection is rare. The symptoms are indistinct and obscure, making it very difficult to identify the cancer until it becomes life threatening.

Today, only 25 percent of ovarian cancers are found before the cancer has spread outside the ovary. At this very early stage, the survival rate is 95 percent and about 90 percent of these women live longer than five years. However, seventy-five percent of ovarian cancers are not discovered until the cancer has spread beyond the ovary. These are the least likely to recover.

"We are fervent advocates of regular gynecologic examinations." She was one of my new doctors from the women's health clinic. "During each examination we will check the pelvic area both internally and externally. Had we seen you before, we would have checked your ovaries and uterus for size, shape and consistency. At least we would have found the tumor before it hemorrhaged. It's always dangerous to operate when a person is in severe trauma. You're a very fortunate woman."

She asked me questions about symptoms prior to the rupture. Did I have abdominal swelling or pressure in the pelvic area?

Or pain in my leg or back or digestive problems like bloating or indigestion? Stomach pain, maybe? What about unusual vaginal bleeding? All of which I had experienced at some point, all of which I ignored. I just never acted on them. I imagined that most women ignored the signs, particularly women competing in the business world.

"Walking," they said when I was sent home to recover, "is the best thing you can do. Walk as much as you can."

It was springtime in Washington and being out among dogwood trees and cherry blossoms was added incentive to go outside. I began walking slowly at first. By the end of my recovery, I was walking over rolling hills in my Sleepy Hollow neighborhood for nearly two hours a day. Unencumbered by work, I was enjoying the exquisite intimacy of being alone with my thoughts. It was then that I began to question the value of my life and wonder about the purpose of my existence. I was in an unhappy marriage, my professional career was stalled, and I felt generally unfulfilled. I clearly remember asking myself, "Don't you get it? This is it." I had often thought that someday I would get to the things that needed changing in my life. I had almost died and that day had never arrived. This was a second chance to get it right.

By summer, I was well enough to return to work, which I did with a new sense of urgency. My near-death experience had caused me to embrace life more fully, to do everything at full throttle. Starting with my career, I began by taking a critical assessment of my life. Assimilating into the corporate system had demanded compromises that, day by day, had resulted in my becoming a small cog in a big machine. I questioned whether or not I made a difference, knowing that I was capable of expanded responsibilities, yet feeling underutilized.

I did not talk about my condition openly and was cautioned that having cancer would taint my promotional opportunities, which I believed were already limited. For me, the stigma of having cancer was significant and I wanted nothing standing in the way of my career. Even among friends, it was a secret.

One day on a business trip shortly after I returned to work, I happened to sit on an airplane next to an older woman who assumed that the time we had together was naturally time for us to visit. I, on the other hand, was attempting to work, undisturbed. The woman, whom I ignored as politely as possible, kept talking as though in a conversation with me. When I finally gave in, she told me she was on a very special trip to see her son.

"I have terminal melanoma." She spoke the words with remarkable calm and I was sorry for being annoyed. But, she was so open and friendly that she had not noticed.

"When I think about dying," she said, "I think that what remains here are the memories people have of you. When I was diagnosed, the saddest part for me was when I realized that the one person in this world who knew me best was a man I really don't love and who doesn't love me, my husband. He knows my habits, the way I think, why I laugh or cry, everything about me. We quarreled all the time and I just don't believe we ever really loved each other. We married young and then we had kids and by the time they grew up and left, we had been together for a long time. I guess we stayed together out of habit, you know how people do. When they told me I had about a year to live, it made me so sad to think that when I am gone, the memory of me will be mostly his. I wish I had been loved deeply by someone who knew me well. Someone special. Those are the memories I would want to leave behind. I decided I should try to end it right, anyway. I left my husband and started spending a few months with each of my children, giving them my last days, showing them how much I love them. I'm on my way to see my son now. I just regret that I didn't do it sooner."

I recall feeling as though we were alone in the airplane—this woman, who was compelled by some unknown force to speak to me, and me. Here we sat like two old friends on a porch having an intimate and private conversation on a sunny afternoon. As she shared her innermost thoughts about life, I realized that I knew too well what she meant, how she felt. It was vivid to me because I was living as she had lived. I decided then to make the changes I was wishing for. I did not think in terms of evolving parts of my life in order to improve existing conditions. I began at the end, deciding what would bring meaning and value to my time on earth and then building the bridge from my current existence to a new reality.

After nineteen years with AT&T, I resigned from my secure position, choosing instead a high-risk venture that led to a senior management position in Oregon.

I then dissolved my marriage.

As each year passed with no indications of cancer, I was convinced that the optimistic prognosis that I had been assured of was correct. I was now cancer-free. An unbelievable gift had been bestowed on me: a gift of a new life. This time it was time to do it right.

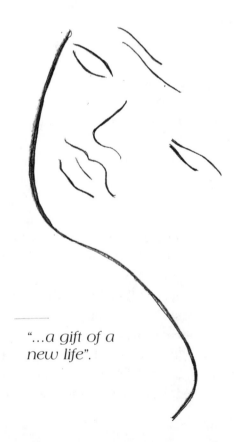

"...a gift of a new life".

7

The Cancer
Persists

Now, twelve years later in my hospital room in Portland, my gynecologist, Dr. Polo, came to tell me that I was no longer his patient because I was being referred to a gynecologic oncologist. This news troubled me. I was uncomfortable about changing doctors at this point and specifically nervous about losing Dr. Polo, who had earned my trust and respect.

"You don't need to be apprehensive. Gynecologic oncology is a highly specialized area of medicine. These are certified, licensed gynecologists who are also trained in cancers specific to the female reproductive system. They have formed a very tight network in order to closely monitor new developments going on throughout the world. You can be very confident that you'll have access to the best medical knowledge available anywhere."

It was reassuring to think that I might finally get answers to the questions about my condition that no one seemed able to address.

"I recommend you see Paul Tseng. He's really the best in this area."

"Whom would you send your wife to?"

"Tseng." He looked me in the eye, not as a patient but as a person.

It was good enough for me. However, it wasn't good enough for my HMO. Dr. Tseng was not directly associated with my medical group and I was asked to consider an oncologist from their list, which I did. Ultimately, the recommendation from Dr. Polo was the deciding factor for me. I presented my case to the HMO over the phone, got support from Dr. Polo and Dr. Van Sickle, and gained concurrence from the carrier to honor the referral. Although this was not the normal appeals process, the matter was handled quickly and professionally.

It had now been a week since my surgery and I was living connected to machines, dismayed that I had more intravenous feeds rather than fewer. In this state of physical and emotional anguish, I began wondering and worrying about what it meant that I had cancer and whether I would live or die. The thought was almost too much for me to process, the implications too much to abide.

One day, a friend who twice had battled breast cancer came to visit. I knew that she could understand me, could know what I feared, could feel what I felt, for she had lived through the same horrendous nightmare not so long ago. She talked, not of the cancer itself, but of the process of living with it, of her emotions and her decisions, of her family and their ability to cope, of thinking it was the worst thing in the world and finding that it was not. And, as a final gift, she gave me a piece of advice that I can still recall with absolute clarity.

"When I went to see the surgeon who I was referred to for a mastectomy, I told him how upset I was at the idea of losing my breast. I was distraught because I felt that it would change me. I just wanted to discuss it with him, to tell him how I felt. But, instead of helping me think it through, he was really abrupt and impatient, as though my feelings were irrelevant because we were discussing life and death issues. Right then I knew he didn't understand me as a person and had no intention of trying to. It was a mechanical problem to him. Or rather, I was a mechanical problem. So, I walked out. The next day I changed doctors because I knew that, regardless of his surgical skills, I could never entrust my life to someone who didn't care about me, the person."

She gave me a perspective that I had not had about my relationship with my oncologist: that together we would be on a long, intimate journey that would last for years. Then she counseled me to find a doctor that I was comfortable with and confident in, one who would listen to me and try to understand me. She was right and I did.

The next day Dr. Tseng came to meet me.

"We just concluded a clinical trial on this particular cancer, granulosa cell. Here's the write-up on it. It's not even published. It's so new that they haven't yet presented the conclusions formally to the AMA."

He handed me seven sheets of paper describing various groups of women who had been in the study, seventy-five women in all. Some, listed as treatment-related mortality, had died from the therapy. The purpose of the trial was to assess the combination of three drugs, bleomycin, etoposide, and cisplatin, as therapy for ovarian stromal malignancies in dosages that would eradicate the cancer cells "while not terminating the patient." It listed various therapies that were used, reporting on the successes and failures. I was struck by the knowledge that so many women had died in the pursuit of an answer to this illness. Each one was someone's wife or mother or daughter. I could have been one of them.

In one group, however, some patients showed significant improvement. The protocol consisted of a particular formula of the three drugs, administered with heavy dosages over twelve weeks. Recurrence was undetermined.

"New clinical trials are being conducted on all types of cancer. We're very lucky this trial was so far along and that it is proving effective on granulosa cell. So, we start therapy as soon as you get home." Tall, with wire-rimmed glasses, Dr. Tseng was serious but excited. He thought we were lucky, but lucky wasn't how I felt right then. The idea of getting well enough to go home so that I could start chemotherapy was very disturbing to me. Even though the pronouncement of an effective therapy was the best news we could hope for, I was scared, angry, and disillusioned. The discovery of an inexorable mass growing inside of me in spite of all the precautions made me feel doomed, as though it was predestined and would always be there. After my first occurrence, I had learned my lessons and was vigilant about check-ups, even nagging my friends, but it hadn't made any difference. I was even tested for tumors a year before but the growth had eluded detection because of its unusual location. The fact that it had returned meant that, statistically, the odds of my survival were greatly diminished. I felt cheated, as though my own body had been deceitful. The sense of loss was hard and real.

More and more, feelings of hopelessness seemed to wash over me. We were dealing with multiple problems and I was having trouble keeping them in order. Rich and I tried to be brave for each other, tried not to think the worst as we saw greater and greater obstacles being erected before our eyes. My faith was faltering. I felt shaken to my very core.

Rich became understandably worried about my emotional state. I was in shock, facing complex decisions with virtually no medical knowledge and was still heavily medicated. For the first time in my life, I was having trouble communicating. I was angry and depressed and very anxious but seemed unable to articulate my feelings because the flood of thoughts and feelings were all jumbled-up inside. One night before Rich went home, he handed me a gift Shirley had sent for Christmas, a big leather-bound journal. Shirley knew how important journals were to me since I had learned about journaling from a good friend and associate, Todd Siler.

When I met Todd a couple of years earlier, I was responsible for leading my company's growth strategies in new business applications. My team was tackling a seemingly unattainable goal: to create millions of dollars in incremental revenue in a saturated telecommunications market. At the same time, Todd had left a teaching position at the Massachusetts Institute of Technology to apply his techniques in interdisciplinary studies to world politics and business. He believed he could open new channels of creative thought by changing the way people think. In his book, *Think Like*

A Genius,[1] Todd describes genius as "thinking of something in a way that no one ever has before." He wrote, "Geniuses are able to see what many miss. They see possibilities in the impossible."

By applying Todd's creative process, my group experienced breakthroughs in new product ideas and market opportunities, exceeding our challenging goals. In the process, not only did I have the benefit of learning from him every time we talked, but Todd and I became good friends.

"I encourage you to always carry a journal. The world is filled with acts of genius and you never know when you might stumble across one. The most amazing, creative, intuitive ideas can come from the most unlikely places."

Once Todd had taught me to use a journal, I was never without one again. "Draw your thoughts," he would say, and I did.

Now, as I lay in the hospital, grappling with my fragmented emotions, my journal began to transform haunting thoughts into shapes or pictures that better expressed my precise meaning with the clarity and intensity I intended but for which there were no words. It became my cache of thoughts, feelings, and dreams. Things I couldn't express verbally, I could draw. Drawings filled the pages, some scary, some hopeful, some soulful. My journal accepted anything. I remember once feeling a sense of betrayal although I couldn't identify exactly why. Then I began to draw. What emerged on the page was a body, my body, being used to nurture a deadly seedling, its branches barren, its roots fused with my blood vessels. I slept better that night.

---

1. Todd Siler: *Think Like A Genius*

"My body, being used to nurture a deadly seedling, its branches barren, its roots fused with my blood vessels".

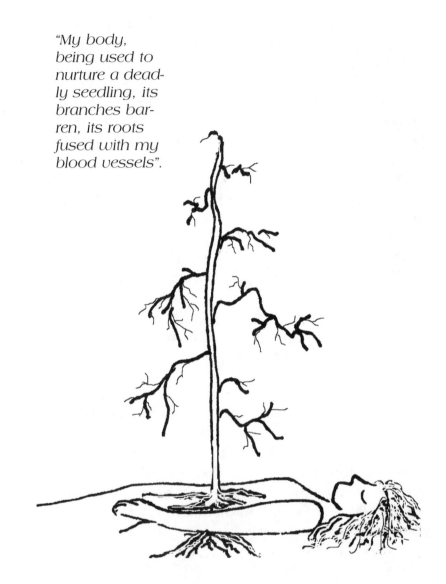

Over the next few days, I began to have an improved grasp of priorities. My first challenge was recovery from the surgery, not cancer treatment. Over the next three weeks, I would expend every ounce of energy to get the fused pieces of my body to function as a system once again. Unfortunately, nothing seemed to be working.

Living in the hospital was getting to me. Sleep was a problem as I was now having drug-induced nightmares on a regular basis. It seemed that I would finally get to sleep when, at about 5:30 every morning, I would be awakened for blood work. The lab technician called it a "vampire visit" because it was taken by attaching a vial to the shunt in my neck, the glass container filling with red liquid touching my face. I could smell it.

"Can't you come later? Surely someone gets blood drawn at seven or eight o'clock."

"No, we like to do our 'vampire visits' first in case there's a problem."

Problem?

He dismissed it and left.

He could do that. In fact, it seemed to me that at any time of the day or night, any medical person could come into my room and do anything he or she wished. This technician was part of a care-giving institution that, while in the daily practice of saving lives, had somehow sacrificed the dignity of the patient in the process. Although it was all for my benefit, I had no choice in their actions, no control of my surroundings. I felt vulnerable and exposed.

At this point Rich was spending as much time with me as possible. He was at the hospital every morning before work, and then he would come again at noon instead of going to lunch. And, of course, every evening after work he stayed until I went to sleep. Every night he would go home, feed our pets, sleep, then return the next day and do it all again. On Saturdays and Sundays he stayed with me all day. He did this for a month.

Outwardly, he was steadfastly optimistic, confident, and strong. But I knew this man and behind the mask I could see the physical and mental exhaustion coupled with his own fears, and I felt awful for causing him so much pain.

Each night his leaving was the time I dreaded most. Not being able to sleep in the comfort of the man I love during the most frightening time of my life was horrible. I knew it was awful for him as well.

One night after he kissed me good night and left the hospital to go home, I opened my journal and wrote:

I miss you. I miss the intimacy of your touch. Your breath at night upon my back as we lie as one in sleep. I miss your smile of tenderness, of gentle loving in all the ways two people can love.

I miss the small signs that everyday give me a million messages of us together. I miss the feel of you — the dance we do in life's little habits. How we move things to make room for eachother. How we change things to accommodate one another. Blending our lives in a way that is - what? harmonic?

I miss having you in my view as I awaken. Talking with you at a meal, being with you, thinking with you, dreaming our dream of dreams with you.

I miss how you make me laugh. I miss how you make me love. I miss you.

8

Living
In The Hospital

Staying in the hospital so long was discouraging and began to break my spirit. For the most part, the medical staff was sympathetic to long-term patients. One nurse, however, did not work well with me for some unknown reason. She seemed unnecessarily rough with some procedures, such as inserting the naso-gastric tube.

The naso-gastric tube, or NG tube, goes into the nose, down through the throat, and into the stomach. Its purpose was to pump out acid. I hated the NG tube. It hurt and it made my throat raw. Simple things, such as talking or sleeping, were painful. Fixated with the idea of getting it out, I made myself believe that the tube was an unnecessary crutch and began disconnecting it for an hour or so—to force my system to deal with the acids on its own. Convinced that I was ready, I had the tube taken out. For the next day and a half, I willed my body to work, envisioning tiny connections lighting up inside. I walked and walked, did breathing exercises, and ignored the nauseous haze that woke me from my sleep. I allowed no other option to enter my mind than that my body was activated. If it were not for this, the buildup of noxious fluids in my reconstructed stomach would cause vomiting. In this case, the NG tube would have to be reinserted.

There was no denying it: the buildup of acids was getting worse, causing me to become increasingly more nauseous by the hour. Still convinced that I could tough it out, I waited until the very last moment in the vain hope that I could change the result. Finally, unable to bear it any longer, I acknowledged defeat. I had wanted it and wished for it but I had failed. Upset that I had lost the battle, I called for the nurse.

"Nurse, I need help. I'm very nauseous."

"You *can't* feel nauseous." She sounded disturbed at me for some reason.

"What do you mean?" I could hardly believe she was correcting me.

"With what you've had done, you can't feel nauseous." She was unyielding.

As she stood there, immovable and annoyed, the dam broke and I began projectile vomiting. Between violent retching I also began to cry from the spasms that seemed to be ripping my stitches apart, gagging in the process. The nurse coolly turned around and left the room. She returned with a new NG tube and another nurse who was to hold me down for the painful reinsertion by forcing the tube back through the nose, down the throat, and into the stomach while I was still vomiting. Rich had to leave the room.

Later, when we learned that I could have been given an anesthetic to relax, which would have facilitated the procedure, Rich met with the head of nursing and asked that other nurses assist me in the future if at all possible. I did not see the calloused nurse again.

We did not ask for or expect special consideration; we simply asked to be respected and listened to. We believed that I had rights as a patient and the hospital agreed. When we had complaints, we voiced our concerns with the management. On the rare occasions when we did have a complaint, we found the hospital administration to be responsive and cooperative.

As the days crawled by, Tracy and her sons became regulars on my floor, often visiting to join me on my afternoon walks. Jonny, the youngest, was fascinated by my new bizarre appendages: curious poles, bags, and tubes. He was no longer nervous in the strange environment and often climbed in bed with me, pushing the controls that adjust the head and feet like some deranged amusement park ride.

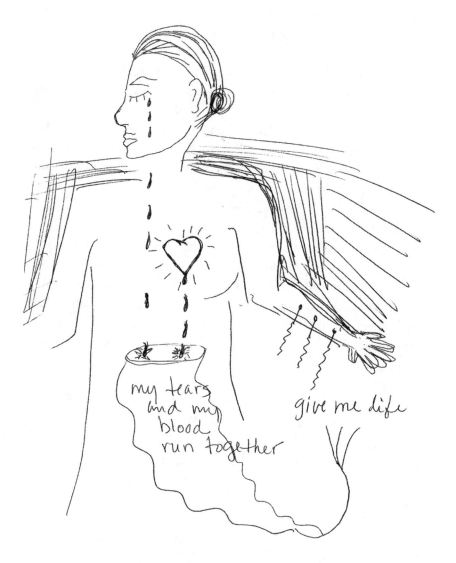

"The nightmares came every night".

Going into the fourth week, the nightmares came every night and they were becoming very weird. In one, I dreamt that I had died. The next morning two nurses came in talking to each other as though I weren't there. All of a sudden, I wasn't sure they could hear or see me and I began to panic. I had been taking morphine for nearly a month, and combining this with the anxiety and stress, I was coming unhinged from lucid, rational thought. At times, I felt on the brink of insanity, unsure of where I was. Twice, I had tried downgrading my pain medication but that induced nausea and tremors, chills, and severe pain. I had failed; I was unable to tolerate removal of the morphine. Worse yet, the drugs exacerbated my feelings of depression. Rich was justifiably worried about my state of mind. Then, he had a brilliant idea.

"I was thinking about calling Dennis."

Dennis Milholm is a psychotherapist whom I had used as a kind of life consultant several years earlier. He had helped me think without the burden of old baggage in order to gain greater clarity about myself in relationship to the world around me. Although I hadn't seen him for a couple of years, my therapy with Dennis had been effective, productive, and healing, as evidenced by how fulfilling and happy my life was now. With my consent, Rich called him right away.

"Why didn't you call me sooner?"

The smile in his blue eyes could not mask the shock of seeing me in my condition. If I hadn't looked so miserable, he would have been angry with me. Instead, he conducted a quick inventory of my medical condition, my current problems, and my mental state.

Yes, I told him, I was in pain at that moment. I had made yet another attempt to decrease my self-administered dosage of morphine.

"I'd like to try hypnosis with you." Dennis had used hypnotherapy in my past sessions. "The most effective use of hypnosis is pain management. We can do it right here, right now."

He moved swiftly, went to the hall and talked to the nurses, and then made a "Do Not Disturb" sign for the door.

He closed the blinds as I closed my eyes. His voice was soft and yet strong against the background noise of the hospital wing. I welcomed the journey. I began floating away from the physical boundaries of my room, away from the clatter in the hall, the disinfectant smell, the voices of people out there who were nothing to do with me. I became light, like a feather, aware of everything, connected to nothing. Dennis's voice guided me through a labyrinth of things familiar, places and faces on the many bridges I had crossed in life.

"You have human potential in you that is untapped. It lives in you and has been waiting for this day. Now you will use it."

Still in hypnotic trance, I arrived at the destination that we sought, one of severed veins and a glut of torn tissues. It was like walking among the rubble after some disaster, except that this disaster was inside of me and it was of me. Yet, I was strangely detached.

"Call on the energy stored within you to flow from all the different parts of your being, and bring it together, and feel it, feel the heat of it. Now send it in search of the damage and command it to begin healing, making thousands of little repairs. The energy is like a laser cauterizing your torn flesh and stopping the torment you feel inside. Your pain is becoming smaller and smaller and it knows it is unwelcome here. Smaller. Your energy hot and alive; it is kinetic with curing powers that flow with your blood through the vessels of your body. The pain is very small now. So small. As the dead cells dissolve away, the pain grows softer . . . softer. You can feel new life in the glow of healing warmth and there is no pain now."

My pain began to fall away as though I were throwing off blankets on a warm summer night, finally finding the breath that had been suffocating underneath. And I could finally breathe. I felt released rather than relieved.

Dennis returned the next day. We talked awhile, and then he put me in a hypnotic trance again. He recorded the hypnosis part of the session so that I could play the tapes to sleep. That night my sleep was deep and restful. I was at peace for the first time in twenty-seven days. It was the last day I took morphine.

By this time, Rich was worn out and needed a break. Then, as though she heard our need, my sister Sylvia took a personal leave

from school and came back to help. Aside from her nurturing attention to my needs, her experience with long-term gastro-intestinal illness caused her to question my situation. She suspected that the
hospital was no longer accelerating my recovery but was now
retarding it. And, she was sure that my loving home and family
were keys to my recovery.

The problem that continued to perplex my doctors was that I
still had no voluntary digestive motility. That meant that I could
not eat because I could not process my food, resulting in my being
fed exclusively by infusion.

"Your machines are all gone with the exception of the intravenous feeding, your pain meds are in pill form, and your only
physical therapy is walking in the hopes that it will jump-start your
guts. I think we should figure out how to do this at home."

With that, Sylvia started investigating rentals of hospital beds
and infusion units and she met with the nurses to discuss taking
over their duties herself. She prayed and she researched. She talked
to God as often as she talked to doctors and technicians. She even
pursued external resources she knew in the field for possible clues
to our dilemma.

One night after she and Rich finally went home, exhausted and troubled, I wrote in my journal the words I could not say.

My Sister

When Sylvia and I were children, I was always her protector. It was my role among us sisters. After all, she was the youngest. Sylvia was my little buddy. I loved being in charge. I could tell her what to do.

Now, as I lie clinging to life, my sister has become my protector. She covers me with a blanket of her love to heal a broken body and fragile spirit. She protects me from the unknown I must face. She stands between my fears and me. I am like a child holding up my hand so that my big sister Sylvia can lead me through the fog of uncertainty, can guide me as I walk along the ledge to arrive where we must go.

It is a precious gift to find my new big sister at this time of my life. To see because of the light she casts on my path so that I will not stumble and fall - knowing that if I do, my sister will lift me up and help me walk again.

One day, I was visited by a beautiful and vibrant woman who had been in and out of chemotherapy for the five years I had known her. I had often wondered how she maintained such a positive outlook while battling breast cancer for several years. Her presence gave me courage, realizing that if she could do it for so long, surely I could do it for four months. Still, I told her I was nervous about chemotherapy and felt overwhelmed.

"That's only natural. Believe me, everyone feels that way. It's not bad enough that you have cancer, now you have to poison your own body to get rid of it. The way to get through it is to not think about the months of chemotherapy ahead of you. Remember that you're going to do it one day at a time. You don't have to do it all today. Just focus on doing one day today. That's all, just one day. And tomorrow, you'll do another day."

She wasn't sympathetic; she was empowering. Most importantly, she was proof that the therapies worked.

"With most medical treatments you feel better soon after the medication is working in your system. With chemo, the exact opposite happens. The treatment makes you sicker. Unfortunately, it works that way. You will get real sick and then you will get better. Remember that. However bad you feel, you will get better. Chemo is hard but for now it's the best we've got. Someday we'll look back on it as barbaric, like some grotesque cure that people endured in the Dark Ages. And there may come days when you think it's too much. But, my only advice to you is this: As bad as it gets, don't think of it as optional. It's our best shot at survival until something better comes along. Chemotherapy can save your life."

Finally, after spending the entire month of January in the hospital and still lacking bowel function, I wondered if the surgery had been too much for the nerves that compose the intricate circuitry of the body. Sylvia, Rich, and I conferred with Dr. Swartz. Was it possible that my organs might never respond?

With Sylvia now trained on my short-term maintenance, we asked Dr. Swartz if I should go home. The doctor wanted to think about it over the weekend.

That Saturday, as Sylvia finalized arrangements for machines to sustain me, the patched-up pieces of my body finally began to function. At long last my intestines were awake. It was an odd thing to celebrate but we did. In fact, we rejoiced as I disconnected myself from intravenous support for the first time in four weeks. I had not eaten food of any kind for a month, but now that I could pass food through my system, I was going home.

9

A Welcome Home

There are no words to adequately express my joy in coming home to familiar surroundings, where the look and smell and taste of my life were mirrored. Now I could kiss Rich good night and close my eyes, safe with the knowledge that when I awoke, I would be in my own bed and lying next to him. I had the sense of something cold inside of me thawing and melting away. I was finally home.

Sylvia spent the next few days getting us organized, doing everything from preparing our kitchen in support of my dietary needs to calling in prescriptions and making doctor appointments. By thinking through the situation, she adjusted things we had not thought of, making our life easier in so many ways. One day she decided to organize my wardrobe for fear of my digging around in my condition. She began by ferreting out any cozy, non-binding clothes, which she then supplemented with a half dozen stretch pants from Target, on sale for $9.99 a pair—a far cry from my accustomed business attire. To those she added tops that buttoned down the front for easy access during infusions, a factor I had not considered. Next, the high heels were culled from the front row and replaced by slippers, flats, and easy-slip-on shoes because bending over to tie laces was impossible. Finally, she inventoried scarves for the time when my hair would be gone. Like playing a kind of reverse dress-up, practical and comfortable were all that mattered now.

"We have to think about what to do when I leave." Sylvia said what we had all been dreading as she dressed my incision. Her life was complicated before my illness, but now things at her home were suffering from her absence. We had delayed it as long as we could because she was an incredible help in so many ways. But, we knew it was time.

"I need to go home soon." And she began checking into flights to return to her four teenagers, her husband, and her classroom.

Although Rich's employer was extremely supportive from the very beginning, they were depending on him to run a business and he had already missed a great deal of work. The only way to manage was with outside help; we needed a caregiver.

Unsure of the available resources, we began pursuing home nursing options through our insurance. Yet, the more we assessed our needs, the less sure we were of how to address them. In my present condition, I required help with virtually everything. More than the medicating and feeding, I needed help to get out of bed, and I could not sit or stand unassisted. I also had numerous medical appointments all over town and required transportation back and forth. And, a stranger in our house would have to deal with our two large dogs. Would we have to kennel our dogs for months if we dropped a new person into their chain of command? One dog was already showing overly protective behavior since my homecoming.

One evening as we discussed our dilemma, William, my sister Carmen's son, came to our rescue.

William had been special to me since he was a little boy. As a child, he had been a devil to discipline but he had the engaging quality of a good boy who just can't help being bad. After he finished high school in Texas, he came to live with me in Virginia because his mother and I thought he needed a major change in his life. Our guess proved to be right and he had grown into a responsible, happy young man. Three years ago, William moved to Portland and was now working at a museum while going to college.

In the hospital, his visits had been anxious. He seemed unable to sit for even a few minutes to talk to me and I could see by the fear in his eyes that he was stunned by my apparent frailty. In some ways he was like a son and I had worried protectively about him, never anticipating that our roles would be reversed.

Since my homecoming, he had visited us every day but he was no longer nervous. He was helping around the house, answering the phone, and talking to us, to them, and to whoever was at the door.

"I'll do it. They're cutting my job to part-time this spring, so I was looking around anyway. I'm not taking classes this semester, so aside from a couple of appointments, I can come over in the morning when Rich goes to work and stay until he's home. Tracy could back me up if we need her. And you just pay me what you can. I'm okay for a couple of months. Besides, you have always supported me when I needed it."

William knew everything about our home and our habits. He had lived with us when he first moved to town and often housesat for us when we were away. Not only could he manage our list of duties, the dogs listened to him and our ancient cat liked him. We knew it was the perfect solution.

"But is it fair?" I wondered if we were exploiting him.

"It's not fair not to accept," Rich's propensity to build character resounded in his logic. "He's part of this family and this is happening to him too. Besides, we need him and it's good for him to be needed. Not only is it important for him to step up; it's important for us to let him."

Thus our family pooled its resources: Sylvia sketched a plan to leave with us that laid out each major area of needs, like meals and meds. William became my primary caregiver on a daily basis, Monday through Friday, and Tracy juggled children, schools, and a supportive husband in order to share chores, including transportation to various clinics or bringing dinner, which she did often. Sylvia, Tracy, and William were passionate about supporting us, not just caring for me but helping Rich to run our lives.

And, Rich, well . . . Who could describe the daily outpouring of love and care, the sense of humor in the face of disaster, the bottomless reservoir of energy. I felt enormous support and love, yet I also felt tremendous guilt. Guilt for bringing pain to my family, scaring them, scaring my mother. Guilt for burdening Rich nonstop for months and adding so much pressure to his demanding business responsibilities. I was troubled because I knew the months ahead would demand the same and more. Much, much more. To make matters worse, I was unaccustomed to having others do virtually everything for me. Dennis and I met again.

"The great psychologists of our time believe that love is the highest goal to which man can aspire. Would you agree?"

Yes. My love for Rich and his for me, and that which we share with our family and friends was healthy and nurturing, whole and real. I was blessed. I had finally found the kind of love that gives meaning to life. Yes.

"These people whom you worry about all love you deeply, each one of them. Don't feel guilty about their feelings. To not want them to have the emotion of loving you to such an extent that they will do anything to help you would be to deny a powerful part of love. You may come away from this experience with a greater love than you even knew you had."

Dennis was right. Tracy was already married and a mother herself when I met her father. She and I grew to like each other easily and smoothly. A beautiful, bright young woman, she was interested in sharing with me a gamut of interests, from literature and art to cooking and personal style. We saw each other often, but we lacked the depth of intimacy that comes with growing up together. Until now. During the months of my illness, Tracy and I became so closely connected that she is as dear to me as though she were my own.

When we met with William to talk about his duties, Rich and I had interpreted his role differently. I still thought of myself as an intelligent, responsible person, competent at managing extensive personal and professional activities. My ability to think had improved since the downgrading of my drugs, and my unusual sleep patterns and intense dreams had faded since I had been home. Generally feeling more stable, I now believed that my limitations were only physical and did not realize how diminished I had become. Naturally, I saw myself as the conductor of an orchestra making all decisions from some comfortable chair, certain that I could figure things out as they arose. I would direct William's activities.

Rich saw William as the decision maker in charge of my care. To begin, he insisted that William manage my schedule of drugs. I thought the suggestion was absurd.

"Really? So, when did you take your last pain pill?" Rich was testing me.

"Ah, about two hours ago . . . I think."

"And, what time is it now?" He was cheating by standing in front of the clock, blocking my view.

"Okay, I don't know," I confessed. I was busted. I really didn't know when I had taken the pill. I had completely lost all sense of time.

"Well, then," Sylvia interjected, "first we need a written schedule for medications. Instead of taking pain meds every four hours, we put specific times that you'll take them every day, like: 8:00 a.m., noon, 4:00 p.m. The times will stay the same but you can vary the amount, maybe taking half of a pill if you don't need as much."

William's first job, then, was to devise a system for administering medications.

Next, we began tracking all medications, procedures, vital signs, appointments, insurance data, and questions for any of the many institutions we would be dealing with, and with whom we had never interacted before. We used our notebook to keep all the information in one place.

"Never get one that is too small," Sylvia warned. "You think a little notebook is great because it's convenient and it'll fit in your purse. But you always lose the little ones, and if you're in a hurry, you don't want to waste time trying to find it."

We began gathering the phone numbers of all the doctors, ther-

apists, nurses, on-call, emergency, hot lines, pharmacies, and on
and on. In a very short time, the floodgate had opened and numbers started appearing from everywhere. Keeping them in one place
was essential.

Eventually, I would be treated in four hospitals plus a cancer
clinic, all in different parts of town. I had eight doctors and interacted with countless nurses. I would have on-call access for out-of-
hours problems and special access numbers for emergencies. There
were day numbers and night numbers and, of course, cell phone
numbers. We would find ourselves communicating daily with pharmacies, labs, outpatient clinics, and insurance representatives from
two carriers. Also, I regularly reported my condition to my company medical department for medical leave approval.

It was also critical that I know not only what procedures were
being performed, but when, where and *why*. We listed which drugs
were being administered, in what dosage, and for what purpose. I
found that the better organized I was and the more articulate about
my condition, the better able I was to ask questions and to verify
any treatment I thought warranted it. As we began building our
own phone book with names, notes, and numbers, Sylvia reluctantly returned to Texas.

One of the hardest things for me to do was to let others do
things for me. I hated being helpless. I didn't want someone else
emptying my dishwasher or fixing dinner in my kitchen. I was
proud of my ability to run simultaneously a family and a business,
too proud. In the beginning, I pushed people away who only wanted to help because they loved me. I was angry about being disabled
and didn't want to be treated like a child. My frustration was often
evident even when I would acquiesce to what needed to be done.

"That's not how I do that."

William was cooking dinner for us with extraordinary patience
while I directed the activity from my chair by the fireplace in the kitchen.

"Get the pan hot before you add the mushrooms." Even as I
spoke them, the words sounded ridiculous, as though culinary technique were the point.

Once, years ago, I was watching a cooking show hosted by the Italian chef, Biba. She spent the entire show preparing an extraordinary bread dish with a surprise filling. Then, in transferring it for final presentation at the table, the bread broke open, exposing the secret within. It had all been for naught. Unflustered, the great chef had laughed a deep, hearty laugh.

"Oh, well," she said easily, "when you make a mistake in the kitchen, remember, it's only food." Yes, I said to myself, it's only food.

Eventually, I would learn to put most things in the context of our recovery mission. Everybody had a job. Mine was to get well; theirs was to help me and sometimes to forgive me. I was learning to be a better patient.

I began to wonder how I could regain command of my life when I had lost control of just about everything in it. As I questioned my ability to impact the crucial matters of major proportion, many annoying little things went unfixed because I didn't care enough to correct them. As an example, my looks were unimportant because of what I had been through over the last few weeks and I was resigned to the fact that things were about to get worse. What difference did it make how I looked now?

While still in the hospital, I had become very frustrated with my hair. My shoulder length hair was drenched from night sweats virtually every night. I was not able to wash it for weeks because of possible exposure to infection around my incision and it was driving me crazy. I tried having the hospital beauty salon "dry wash" it–a horrible mistake. One day, out of desperation, I stood at the hospital sink and started cutting my own hair. As word spread down the wing, nurses came to gawk at the bizarre sight. It had given me a definite punk–like quality, with tufts of chopped hair sticking up everywhere. Now that I was home and feeling lucky just to be clean, I abandoned any effort to fix it.

As a corporate executive with several community and arts boards appointments, I routinely attended numerous formal events and business functions. For ten years, the same hair stylist, Roxanne, had coiffured me for them all perfectly. In those days I would bring in ball gowns or couture suits, trusting her alone to design my then-considerable mane. She styled my hair for my wedding and for every other important event. I had spent many hours in her chair and in the process we had become great friends. One day, shortly after I had returned home from the hospital, she called to check on me.

"Would you like me to come over? Maybe I could cut your hair for you?"

"I suppose Rich told you I cut it in the hospital," I said, trying not to sound self-pitying. Rich, her second favorite client, had reported to her on my progress.

"Well, he said you used those little scissors that are for cutting stitches." She was laughing at the mental image of me in a hospital gown at the sink, hacking away at my gnarled locks. The days when she had designed the hair to the costume were a long-distant memory.

"I'm coming out tomorrow. Let's just see what I can do."

It seemed ridiculous, having Roxanne leave the salon for a couple of hours and travel across town to see me. What difference did it make now?

When she arrived the next day, the actual sight of my hair was apparently as amusing as the mental image had been.

"Go ahead and laugh. Pretty soon I won't have any hair. Then how are you gonna buy groceries? Think about that when you're laughing at me," feigning insult while glad to see my friend.

"When your hair goes, I think we should dye your scalp like body art." Roxanne acted genuinely excited. "Wouldn't that be great? I saw this new henna product and I'm going to order it. Come on! It'll look really hip."

I laughed out loud for the first time in much too long. Roxanne always makes me laugh and, although it hurt, for a couple of hours we did anyway. We had lunch and Roxanne repaired what she could of my hair, vowing to come back even when it was gone. In the months that followed, although we never dyed my scalp, I would look forward to her visits because they helped me restore my connection with the body that I felt had deceived me in a thousand conversations every single day for over a decade.

I continued to see Dennis for help with feelings I did not understand, like the waves of resentment that seemed to be growing stronger.

"Tell me what goes through your mind when you feel this way." Dennis began drawing the drape we put on the uncomfortable.

To me it did not seem fair. After all, weren't there horrible people in the world? Why wasn't this happening to them instead of me? I tried to live right. I had a good life that was hard won; nothing had come easily. Why this? Why now? What was God thinking?

"You sound as though you have earned the right to a certain life that is being taken away from you unjustly. You're applying principles that have no validity here. It doesn't really matter what you expect from life. What matters is what life demands from you. So, basically, you must make some decisions. How do you choose to deal with what life has now dealt you? Don't look to God for answers. Look to God to give you the wisdom to look within yourself."

Dennis's approach to my therapy was based on a philosophical belief that we, as human beings, are driven by our ability to reason and that our motivation is to find purpose and meaning for our existence. This approach to therapy is based on the foundation of a psychological doctrine known as "logo therapy." "Logos" is Greek for "meaning" and refers to the theories that emerged from the Third Viennese School of Psychotherapy in the second half of the twentieth century. This school, focused on "the meaning of human existence as well as on man's search for such meaning," is more concerned with determining the future rather than reliving the past.

The foremost authority and founder of these studies in human behavior was a Holocaust survivor, Viktor Frankl, who taught psychiatric studies in Vienna when Hitler invaded Austria. In his book, *Man's Search For Meaning*,[1] he recounts his experience in concentration camps for three years not as a doctor but as a prisoner. It is with remarkable perspective that he describes the dimensions of human existence under horrific conditions.

---

1. Viktor Frankl: *Man's Search For Meaning*

"Frankl observed man being stripped down to a primitive form of mental health through physical torture, nutritional starvation, and psychological loss of dignity," Dennis explained, handing me the book. "This man was a brilliant, world-renowned doctor and educator. When the Jews were being targeted in Europe, he was invited to immigrate to America. Instead of saving himself, he chose to stay with his family and thus became a prisoner. Finding himself in this unfortunate position, he then decided to use it as a laboratory in which to study man in extreme conditions. He observes from both sides the elements of humanity that allow one group of people to completely dehumanize another. In his remarkable writings you'll find that beyond his observations of man's capacity to destroy, he discovers new truths about man's capability to survive. That's where your lesson is."

I learned about Frankl's examining the effect of shattering the family structure and its impact on the psychological and physiological health of the individual. As I read how the Nazis had strategically broken the spirit of the people by breaking the bonds with their loved ones, I was humbled by the abundant love and support that surrounded me.

The main conclusion about human behavior in Frankl's book is that the one distinguishing factor that determines our existence under harsh conditions is the "will to live." Even his own survival became tied to his commitment to publish his findings and tell the world of his ghastly, horrific experiences and observations.

It surprised me that Frankl didn't believe it mattered whether the goal is altruistic or not; the result was the same. Those who had a reason to live seemed to defy death. He cites numerous examples of prisoners enduring the most unimaginable brutality under deplorable conditions, surviving because some inner force drove them to do so.

"This is what we refer to as the psychology of your illness. It has to do with your deeper unconscious beliefs and feelings and the incredible influence they have on your very physiology."

Dennis demonstrated this connective response with an exercise, having me relax with my eyes closed, and visualizing a large, yellow lemon. I imagined myself cutting the lemon in half, seeing the juice of the ripe fruit run down the slice as I cut into it. In my mind I lifted it to my lips, smelling the acidic essence as I imagined biting into it, tasting the sourness invade my mouth, and I begin to salivate from a lemon that wasn't there.

Next we employed a technique known as visualization, pinpoint concentration on the revitalization of healthy cells. This process demanded that I simplify my thinking in order to apply the full force of my being on healing, and in the process, let go of negative feelings, such as self-pity, as liabilities. Dennis facilitated this process with the use of hypnosis, which he based on the teachings of Dr. Milton Erickson, considered by many to be the greatest innovator and teacher of therapeutic hypnotherapy.

"There is a world of difference between the use of hypnosis for psychotherapy and using it for entertainment." Dennis described Erickson's philosophy and the principles of his teachings.

"Erickson's approach begins with a belief that each and every person is unique, with unique thoughts, behaviors, actions, and reactions. We must first understand a person's uniqueness and appreciate it on its many levels, levels we attempt to reach through the unconscious."

Dennis had often shared with me his belief that people have far more abilities and resources than we are aware of consciously. He also believes that a person's unconscious can act independently of the conscious.

"We don't need to think consciously about certain things for the body to decide to do them, like breathing or sleeping. That's the unconscious part of your brain making decisions and causing things to happen. Hypnosis is a way for us to reach the unconscious, to communicate with it so that we can access those hidden resources."

Our goal was mastering the integration and cooperation between the conscious and unconscious with hypnotic trance. This approach was more concerned with finding ways to achieve my current needs and goals, and less with understanding the past. My sessions focused on moving forward and provided me the tools to arrive there. During these sessions, Dennis would lead me into trance with stories filled with symbols and signs, helping me see from a new perspective. Regardless of the subject of the story, I always sensed that he was talking to me, about me, pointing out things, showing and teaching me. I would hear his voice clearly telling me to "remember to remember," the phrase that triggers me to summon memories from my deep subconscious; to "forget to remember," releasing me from counterproductive memories, such as recalling the pain or fear of treatments, and finally to "remember to forget," my weapon to dispatch burdensome negative thoughts.

For me, trance was natural, calming and yet energizing and empowering. Afterward I always felt rested and peaceful. In trance, I chose to open doors that were useful and productive, and I "walked" past those that were not. I had choices about how to approach my life, cancer and all.

An important part of our work was the development of tools to tap the immeasurable power of my emotions. I already believed in the need for healthy emotions in achieving personal depth and inner strength. Now, we went a step further by looking at the energy associated with rage, for example, as fantastic energy that could assist in my healing. When feelings of anger began to emerge, Dennis helped me redirect my feelings, not by diminishing their intensity, but by approaching anger as an energy source that had yet to find the right channel.

"Is fire good or bad? The answer's 'both' and the answer's 'neither' because it depends on precisely how you use it. So, you get to decide how to use energy created by intense emotion."

In trance, I envisioned harnessing the powerful energy and dispatching it to tasks needed to give my body new vigor.

Dennis began laying a psychological foundation with a mindset where recovery would be my goal and I would be continually focused on it. He further helped me rediscover times from my past when I had gone very deep inside for the strength to overcome seemingly insurmountable obstacles. They had been my training for this moment of my life.

Through therapy, I gained a stronger spiritual and psychological base to endure a condition that often damages both very deeply. My sessions helped me attain a stable mindset of health which began with my thinking of my "problem" in terms of "problem solving."

I was scheduled to begin chemotherapy two weeks after my release from the hospital and my physical condition at the time was not good. After a month of being fed intravenously, I had lost weight and was very weak. The fourteen-inch incision down the front of my torso was healing but still angry and painful. However, the fact that my cancer had returned and that it was not isolated to reproductive organs meant that cancer cells were probably still living in me and could emerge at any time, anywhere in my body. Although the tumor had been removed, Dr. Tseng wanted to begin chemotherapy right away.

"I think I need more time, Dr. Tseng," I pleaded ineffectively. "I'm still pretty messed up from the surgery. Can I have a month before we start?" I was afraid.

"Absolutely not! Look, we really don't want to delay this. These cells are microscopic, so they could be anywhere in your body. We need to get to them now while there's a better chance of killing whatever's in your system. Besides, this way you'll have all this behind you by summer."

My digestive process was not yet stable and any number of things could upset it. On my release from the hospital, the nurse didn't have specific instructions about food and when I asked her about diet, she just imparted her general advice, assuming it would be best for me. She gave me suggestions of tolerable foods such as soft, plain foods with minimal roughage. No one discussed nutrition, just calories.

"You'll find that some foods will move through you more quickly," she said, "so, you should add richer foods to your diet to keep your calorie count up. Try drinking Ensure between meals."

Another remarkable connection occurred when I met Joanne Leyva at my gym the previous summer. Joanne had been an administrator at a VA hospital until she decided to shift gears and pursue her passion for physical fitness. She became a personal trainer with an emphasis on overall wellness. One day, she came to visit and her nursing background painted a vivid picture of how challenging the obstacles ahead would be, particularly because of how weak my body was becoming. She tried to be encouraging even though intuitively I knew she was afraid for me. She took notes of my medical condition, promising to come back with suggestions to help me. I did not know then that Joanne would be key to my survival, and that in the long and difficult months that followed, she would devise the strategy to optimize my body's resources and produce the energy for fierce combat.

Joanne could see that I moved with great difficulty, hunched over from the incision that extended the length of my torso, healing in such a way as to draw me into a fetal position. Feeling lucky to be eating anything, I had not wanted to upset my system if at all possible. Therefore, my "diet" consisted mostly of toast, potatoes, pasta, and soup. As Joanne and I discussed this, her concern intensified because she feared that my meager attempts at nourishment were being compromised by a gastrointestinal system that minimized the time available for nutrient absorption. I was probably extracting little of the value of the limited foods I was offering to my system.

"This is more serious than you realize. You are about to start chemo and that is going to deplete your reserves even further. Your digestion is not efficient and you're losing weight too fast. Plus, when the body is healing, it uses additional energy. The way things are going, you won't have any resources left and your body will literally start eating itself for fuel. How much weight have you lost since this all started?" She frowned as she helped me get out of bed.

"Twenty-five pounds in five weeks," like an infomercial for a miracle diet.

"Too much," she warned, shaking her head. "It's too much, too soon. We're so focused on being thin that we think all weight loss is good. It's not. Let me tell you what's going on with your body. You've been in a hospital bed with virtually no activity for a month, fasting the entire time. Now, on a bland, high calorie diet, your body is dumping most of what it takes in, including vitamins, nutrients, and even anti-carcinogens that occur naturally in food. A lot of the weight you're losing is your body cannibalizing its own muscle tissue to feed itself."

Joanne's passion and training converged into her beliefs that nutritional status and healing are inextricably tied to one another.

"Think of the process the body goes through healing itself: building new tissue, fighting infection, making new blood. These are all serious consumers of energy, energy created by burning fuel. We need to give your body the resources to create that energy and optimize your ability to endure chemo without retarding your healing requirements in the process. I know that nutrition is the key here."

Joanne decided to work up some nutritional recommendations for me. Then, she asked the impossible. She suggested that I get up and move every day.

"Think of it this way. If you were preparing to run a marathon, you'd train for it. Every day you'd be strengthening your body, improving your stamina, making your systems as fit as possible to sustain you during the event. Well, this is the most important marathon of your life, and the same principles apply. The difference is that you're asking your body to perform under exceptionally tough conditions over a long period of time. You've already burdened yourself by depleting your physical resources. Now, you have to be as fit as possible as you go into the next few months—so that you can succeed. Give your body the very best chance it has to win."

She knew then—but I really did not comprehend—that the worst was still ahead. Later, Joanne would tell me of trying to conceal her fear that I would die, unable to endure the ravages of chemotherapy. In the last five weeks my body had been wasting and it had yet to begin the long battle to save itself.

As the time to begin chemotherapy grew near, I became more and more nervous. I had no idea what the full impact would be when we began pouring toxins into my body. It was hard not to feel frightened. Dennis came to get me mentally prepared.

"Your soul and your spirit are healthy and strong, and that is the essence of you: what is in your mind and your heart. Not this body. Unfortunately, your body is a shell that's defective and you need to get it fixed, that's all. Sure, it will be long and difficult, but it's one of those things you have to do now, because that's what it'll take to get you well again. Just remember that whatever the treatments are doing, they are not doing to you but to the thing outside of you, the housing for your true self."

My anti-cancer drugs would be administered by infusing chemicals into the heart via a shunt or access port which would be installed in my chest. I selected a "port-a-cath" because it was fully embedded into the body and would allow me to have baths and showers without concern of infections. It would, however, require a needle stick each time I received daily infusions. Day surgery to install the port was scheduled the week before beginning chemotherapy. All the while I tried to ignore my dread of going back for even a simple procedure.

Then, I got some great news. Knowing that returning to the hospital would be difficult for me, my friend Shirley was coming from Washington to take me in for the surgery. She had called every day while I was in the hospital, attempting to close the distance between us through daily contact. With me, she was happy, upbeat, and enthusiastic; the painful conversations were between her and Rich away from my earshot. The day she arrived she walked into our kitchen to hug me but on seeing me barely able to stand, weak and small, she could not mask her agony.

"Oh my god, Annette, I wish I could have been here sooner." And she cried.

But she had been here. I showed her the journal, her gift to me the day before I became ill, the journal that now kept my very deep secrets, like any best friend. And we talked into the evening about love and life and the meaning of both.

The next morning Shirley drove me in the cold drizzle to the hospital for the outpatient procedure. As we sat waiting, Shirley reminisced about our learning together to swim in the dangerous waters of corporate America. Beyond intelligence and experience, it had taken sheer strength to stay in the game.

"I remember once you had to be in a different city every day for two weeks to roll out the new business strategy. There you were hopping from town to town, schlepping around all this marketing data, making presentations to thousands of people. It's incredible that you didn't end up in the hospital then. But you didn't. You just kept on going."

"Actually, those days were fun. The real test was staying up all night generating endless reports to satisfy the corporate lust for information. The trick is finding the energy to do things you don't want to do."

The surgery was to be performed by Dr. Swartz and before we began, he came to speak with me, explaining his expectations of the morning.

"I want to position the device as close to the heart as possible because that's where the infusions are going. I think that the farther you get from the target, the greater risks you introduce. We do this surgery all the time. I've scheduled it for twenty minutes assuming we don't run into complications."

However, it was two hours later that Dr. Swartz resolved a problem in securing the port to my chest muscles. My body was determined to make him work for everything. After attempting installation in several locations, he finally secured the device to the left pectoral tissue at an odd angle. We did not know then but would soon discover that this would prove to be a challenge every day that I received infusions in the months ahead.

Shirley took me home, put me to bed with pain medication, and made dinner. That night we talked.

"While you were in surgery I kept thinking about how you used to sign us up for these Herculean tasks, and I would think, 'How are we going to do that? We've never done that before.' You would just laugh and say, 'So what? No one is born an expert. Everybody starts at the beginning.' And when I would doubt myself, you would tell me to just believe, 'believe in yourself and others will believe in you.' When I leave tomorrow, I want to leave you with those thoughts from my teacher—you."

Shirley is one of three women who are my best friends. The other two, Zelda and Dayna, had been my friends for over twenty years, friends I met when I moved to California in the late seventies. They had been in almost daily communication with us and with each other from the beginning and worked out a schedule so that as one left, another would arrive. Professional women with enormous responsibilities, they set aside their other commitments to come to Portland to help. Coincidentally, each had recently lost a friend to cancer. They did not want to lose another.

Zelda and I met in 1978, at a time when I was assigned to manage communications at NASA Ames and Sunnyvale Air Force Base, a sophisticated command and control facility. It was the genesis of the space shuttle program and my responsibilities required a great deal of precision and security. Working hard to establish credibility in the male-dominated defense industry, I had developed disciplines that had been lacking in the execution of the contract I was now managing. As an extension of my duties, I was also chairing a conference that was a joint effort between industry and the military. It was "my baby."

Zelda worked for another contractor who was involved with satellite technology and was assigned to facilitate communications among the principals of her company and the commanding officers of the U.S. Air Force Space Command.

One day, while walking down the hall of the secure complex, I was startled by a shout from the far corridor. The colonel who was my military contact had spotted me, yelled out my name, and excitedly flagged me down.

"Guess what!" he was effusive. "I've found someone to take on part of the program. Isn't that great?"

My program?

"Oh, she's so terrific. Just wait till you meet her. I told her to come to your meeting and you'd put her on the team." The colonel was smitten, I could tell.

"I really appreciate your help but don't you think we should have discussed it before you talked to her?" I attempted to mask my agitation that my authority had been usurped. I tried to make my point tactfully because the situation was delicate.

"No problem. Just wait till you meet her. Her name is Zelda and I know you'll just love her!"

He didn't get it. But, he was my customer and his actions were well intentioned. There was, however, no doubt in my mind that I would not "love" Zelda. At that moment I was working hard not to hate her and had yet to even meet her. She came into the meeting later that afternoon, breezy and sweet and attractive. I decided to probe so that I could assess her, ferret out those weaknesses I knew she had. What I got in return disarmed me. She was the most open person I had ever met or have met since. By the end of the meeting, I was smitten with her as well; we all were.

Zelda and I did collaborate on the project together, working like crazy to make our program wildly successful, which it was. At that time we were working with the pioneers of the satellite and space shuttle programs. We interacted with extraordinary thinkers and builders, scientists and engineers. And, we were in Silicon Valley when huge changes were creating a revolution in the computer industry. It was thrilling. We were playing on the edge of the blade and loved it.

Zelda grew so much during the experience that she struck out after that and started a public relations agency on her own. Later she married a wonderful guy who joined her in building one of the top agencies in the country. We saw each other often over the years and had remained close while I moved from coast to coast.

"I'm coming Wednesday! I'm so excited to see you." She had arranged her arrival in Portland to coincide with Shirley's departure.

"When I get there we'll have to do something crazy! What do you think? Do you think Richie can handle it?" She is always effervescent. It is a state of being with Zelda. Once, she and I met another friend at a spa in Mexico. The other friend and I were veterans and assumed we would be leading Zelda around. Within two days, without knowing how it happened, the tables had turned. In every class, when we introduced ourselves to other guests, we were met with, "Oh, you're the friends of Zelda." She is a rare combination of tax auditor and Tinker Bell. I could see fairy dust coming through the receiver as she spoke. "I know! We'll have a little party to celebrate your release from the hospital. Can you have champagne?"

"Oh, yeah . . . right, Zelda, a party was exactly what I had in mind." I shuffled around the kitchen with the cordless phone, struggling to stand up straight, chuckling at the absurd suggestion. I wondered if she would be wearing a cheerleader outfit on the plane and how Rich would react to it. Nothing would surprise me.

She wasn't in costume but she was toting bundles and bundles of the most outrageous socks to be found in San Francisco. A perfect gift. A voracious reader herself, she also brought books, lots and lots of books. Novels, spiritual books, books on healing and feng shui. And, of course, this amazing inner light that she emits, beaming with the same intensity as it has for the twenty years I had known her. Her beautiful long arms embraced me like a sister and we laughed and cried; we had been through so many life changes together and now we faced another, terrible and frightening and cold.

"Tell me everything, everything. I want to know it all." She would intensify her empathy by reliving my pain and anguish. For the next couple of hours she took it all in and I had the reaction of lessening my load. Just a few rocks fell out of the sack that I carried and I felt better. The powerful magic of friendship was working.

"I think we should do something fun. Come on, let's go for sushi!" Just like that, the same as it has been for years, a familiar pas-

time. Now it was time for a party. Zelda's ability to rally was leg-
endary and she was famous for bringing out the excitement genes
in everyone around her.

"Sushi's a quantum leap from mashed potatoes, Zelda." Painful
as it was, I was laughing again. This could be exciting.

"So? We won't know unless we try, right? You think a little raw
fish is going to kill you after what you've been through? Be real!
Sushi always fixed anything that ever bothered us before, from split
ends to split marriages. I say we do it."

How could I refuse? I wouldn't know where to start the argu-
ment, which I believe is the secret to her success.

With that, Rich took us to a neighborhood sushi bar and, for
the first time in a long time, it felt great to get out. At dinner, we
began reliving our adventures, laughing about the fun and the
foibles, revealing to Rich all of our zany recollections. Then, like a
magic movie projector, I was lost in the story of two young women
two decades ago.

The next morning Zelda came to my room and sat on the bed
to talk to me. I could tell by the look in her eyes that she had been
up most of the night.

"Talking at dinner last night brought on a rush of memories
from that time in my life when we first met. You know, I had never
really been on my own before. I was married right out of school and
for all my life, up to that point, someone made all the major decisions for me. Then, when we worked together, I felt responsible and
respected and self-assured. All this unleashed power was intoxicat-
ing and it made me think I could do anything. So, I split from a
bad marriage although I had no place to live. Then I quit my job
because I had this dream to start a business, even though I didn't
really have a business plan. I can't believe I severed all my support
systems at once. How naive I was! But, what I did have was the confidence to succeed. And, when I got nervous about whether I could
do it, I thought, 'Annette thinks I can do it, so I guess I can.' And,
I did."

The tears ran down her face but her voice never faltered. She had become a remarkable woman.

"So I got up this morning and realized that even though this seems terrifying right now, I know that you're going to conquer it. There's no question in my mind that you will look back on your battle with cancer as one more achievement in your life. That's all it is—an achievement in the making. I am so confident about it that I'm not afraid anymore. I'm sorry that it has to be so hard for you but I know that in the end, you're going to prevail." I considered her thoughts as she helped me out of bed and got me dressed for a short walk. She supported me physically as if helping an aged parent, but with the love between friends who see perfect beauty in each other.

Zelda went home the day Dayna arrived.

Dayna and I had worked together in the Bay Area in 1981 at the time of the divestiture of AT&T. I met her the first day of business of American Bell, a new mega-corporation created by the breakup of the Bell System. We were chosen to be part of a new unregulated, competitive sales machine, selected through a stringent two-year assessment process. Those drafted for the new business had proven skills in professional account management; we were students of our craft. She was ten years younger than I so I knew she must be smart to make the team. She was.

Fresh out of Berkeley, she had "fast tracked" into an account executive position and was working aggressively to master the necessary competencies for success. It would not take her long. To this day I consider her the only person I would be afraid to compete against. She is directed and strong, disciplined and focused, and very quick. She takes no prisoners.

When we met in Oakland, we became instant friends.

"Annette, I had to be your friend. You kept parading men in uniform through the office." A standing joke for years about my military clients.

For the two years we worked together, Dayna and I became each other's sounding board, debating politics or business or technology. I marveled at her rapid development, her only limitation—her lack of experience. If she had done it once, whatever it was, she knew how to do it right. She learned everything the first time. She never could understand why others did not.

When I moved back east, our friendship actually became closer. Distance was never an issue because we routinely traveled cross-country and were able to visit each other several times a year. We enjoyed many of the same things and always appreciated them more when we were together. About the time of my subsequent move to Oregon, Dayna left California, opting for Arizona sun instead. In recent years, Rich and I visited her often during our rainy season.

Her arrival was timed so that she could take me through chemotherapy orientation on Friday, and then on Monday stay with me for my first day of infusions.

"I'm stunned that this is happening to you. I just can't believe that there were no warning signs, no symptoms, no nothing until—BOOM—just like that, 'I'm sorry, but you have cancer and you're probably going to die.' How does that happen?" She was angry, disbelieving. I knew that look. She wanted answers.

Dayna, like many people, had read news articles describing advances in cancer screening and early detection. Her direct knowledge of the disease, however, was limited to the experiences of people close to her who had become ill.

"Why didn't they know this before? What kind of tests have they been running all these years? Don't they check you regularly for cancer? I just don't get it."

The prior year, after experiencing sharp abdominal pains, I had undergone an ultrasound for the specific purpose of looking for tumors, but none had shown up on any tests.

"They couldn't even identify it as cancer when I was in the hospital until they removed it. They ran test after test but couldn't tell what it was until the lab performed a biopsy. You know, we're a long way from fool-proof cancer screening." I depicted my understanding of the elusive nature of the tumor I had spawned, hoping I would not have to write a report.

"It's just frustrating that you can do everything you're supposed to and still end up here . . . or worse," her words divulging an exasperation that I shared.

In the end, she was assuaged by the knowledge that we had made sound choices under the guidance of great doctors, and that we were fully invested in the treatment plan that was laid out for me. We believed that we were doing all that could be done to alter the course on which I had been launched.

Like Shirley and Zelda before her, Dayna came, not to soothe my wounds, but to begin filling a reservoir of courage I would use again and again during my battle. We four friends were different in the ways one commonly groups people: personality, background, and lifestyle. Yet, we shared a common fervor, not to merely survive, but to thrive in our particular universe. At some point in our past, we had learned together to overcome life's barriers and achieve happiness. Each in her unique way came to remind me of our large and small triumphs, resolute in her belief that the power to realize them had come from within and, with tested grit and pure sincerity, had opened her heart to me, imbuing me with feelings of being both more empowered and yet more peaceful at the same time.

I opened my journal and wrote words that hungered for the page.

My Friends

I am your friend and you are mine. We chose eachother so! Did I choose you because of what you reflect in me? Is our friendship a special place where we can laugh or cry unlike with anyone else? Do you find something special about yourself when we're together as I do?

Friendship. Where does it start? Where does it end? Can you feel the warmth of it? Can you touch it and know its strength?

It is human loving without conditions, without boundaries. Friendship draws from us that which we wish to be and mirrors it in the face of another.

I may not be everything you think I am. I may forget, mistake, confuse or complicate. I might drop the ball,... I may not see it at all. But I am and always will be your friend.

Your reflection of me or mine of you can be pristine. It is, after all, made of love and dreams and memory dust. What is perfect is our friendship. It is unique, the one and only friendship between us, a bond with none other.

"I'll be there for you," so our friendship says. And so you are. So you always have been and I know you always will be. Because you are my friend. And I love you for it. And I'll be there for you.

10

Chemotherapy

On Friday morning, we arrived at Northwest Cancer Specialists for orientation where we met with Dr. Tseng to review his treatment strategy. He said that since my cancer had recurred after twelve years, we should assume that I was still hosting cancer cells in other tissues of my body. Until very recently, there had been no effective chemical combination to treat the disease, which was the reason I had not been given chemotherapy with the earlier occurrence. Now, at the conclusion of multi-year clinical trials, oncology could offer a new weapon in the battle with ovarian cancer: deadly doses of chemicals to kill any remaining cancer cells. The doctor summarized the clinical aspects of my chemotherapy protocol, the particular dosages and treatment modalities, explaining that the treatment would be intense, but that it had proved effective in improving the five-year survival rate of ovarian cancer patients.

"There are a number of side effects which we'll go over with you in detail later. Is there anything I can answer for you now?"

I had no frame of reference for this situation, completely out of my element and at a loss as to what questions to ask. I said nothing.

"Most women want to know about the hair. Well, you will lose your hair with this therapy, but don't worry. It will come back."

I could only rely on my confidence in Dr. Tseng and assumed

that his knowledge and skill were all that mattered. I would put myself completely in his hands.

Once Rich left for work, Dayna accompanied me to the in-depth orientation where she took copious notes, keeping endless details straight for me to digest later when the shock of the experience wore off.

"You will be very busy," the nurse told me as she handed me a schedule for the next three months, broken down into three-week cycles. Every box on the calendar had notes in it. "Every day for a week, starting Monday, you'll come here for infusions which will last five to six hours."

"Five to six hours?" I wasn't sure I had heard correctly. "I'll be getting infusions for five to six hours? That's all day. What happened to 'go to chemo in the morning, go to work in the afternoon?' I had no idea it was all day." I felt disoriented at the unexpected news.

"The drugs you're taking are highly toxic, so the infusions are administered slowly with other fluids. You see, chemotherapy isn't the same for everyone. In fact, 'chemotherapy' is a generic term for treatment using anti-cancer drugs. Each kind of cancer has a different combination of drugs, given at different intervals, and some are even administered differently. It's true that some patients come in for an hour or so and then go about their business, leading relatively normal lives. Some even take the drugs in pill form. But, in your case we need a concentrated dosage in order to be effective. That's why hydration is so important. Not only will you need fluids to carry the drugs into your system, we don't want one of the drugs, Cisplatin, sitting in your kidneys where it could do some damage. On infusion days, you'll be with us pretty much all day. Now, the next week . . ."

The nurse practitioner kept talking but I didn't hear her. I had begun to weep, the reality of it all squeezing my spirit into submission. The hospital didn't break me, but maybe this would. I felt drenched in misery. I had never imagined myself here.

"I'm sorry, Annette. It's a lot, isn't it? Do you need some time?"

Her concern was genuine.

"No . . . no, I'm all right." Regaining control. "What did you say about the next week?"

"For the next week and a half you'll go to Meridian Park Hospital for injections to regenerate your red and white blood cells. Your anti-cancer drugs lower the red and white blood count by suppressing your bone marrow. The shots help rebuild your immune system." Dayna scribbled while I tried to steady my breathing.

"You'll be susceptible to infection so it's important to take your temperature twice a day. If it's over 100.4 degrees, call in. There, on your calendar you'll see 'Labs' several times. Those are the days we draw blood to see if you're missing anything, and then on the weekends, you'll get infusions to hydrate you and add whatever you need. You'll go to St. Vincent's for those treatments."

"What about these three boxes?" I spotted three days at the end of the cycle without annotations.

"Those are your days off."

Eventually, we came to the discussion of side effects.

"There will be reactions to these drugs, since they work by killing all the fast growing cells, both good and bad. The body has no way to distinguish between the two. Remember that all the side effects are temporary. Typically, they include nausea and vomiting, lack of hunger, pain around the injection site, fatigue, chills, weakness, tingling of the hands and feet, being tired or confused, rashes, redness and tearing of the eyes, diarrhea or constipation, and hair loss. However, chemotherapy has no impact on your sex drive. You should just continue your regular patterns." The statement seemed somewhat incongruous.

"We'll give you several medications to help manage nausea, pain, and insomnia. If you have any other problems, let us know right away. After hours, call the all-night service and ask for a nurse. You'll also be hypersensitive to the sun, so use adequate skin protection and try to limit your exposure with hats and protective clothing. The treatments can tend to dry out your skin so we recommend using soaps and lotions without perfumes or alcohol. No dental work without telling the doctor; in fact, nothing that might expose your blood. The decrease in platelet count means you'll have trouble with blood clotting, so we need to be careful about bleeding. And, generally, do whatever you can to control your exposure to germs, contagious disease, or anything else that could make you ill. The natural defenses of your body are severely inhibited during chemotherapy."

I was taken to the treatment room where I would spend the next few months getting my injections. The walls were lined with recliners, each occupied by a cancer patient. Some were sleeping, some eating, some throwing up. It made me dizzy realizing that Monday I would be one of them. And, I could not get over the shock at finding that something I considered so personal would take place out in the open, with no privacy at all. I had not expected it. Instantly, I was fifteen again, standing in a cancer ward in Houston, only this time I was not looking for my father's bed but for my own. At that moment I felt dizzy, as if I were in a free fall.

Since my stay in the hospital, I had felt powerless, reacting to things that were happening to me. In that first month, I had been poked and probed, handled by countless medical people, any time of day or night. There had been no choices for me then and there seemed to be none now. I was stepping from one nightmare into another, trying to hold myself together but inside on the verge of despair. It was then that I broke down. I thought I was in hell.

Sunday was Valentine's Day and Rich gave me flowers and a beautiful scarf and new satin slippers. He fixed a simple dinner while Dayna returned dozens of business messages to allow her to be away with me the next day. I tried not to think about the morning, but I was so thankful that Dayna would be going with me. Then, too soon, the evening was coming to an end. Before going to bed, Dayna made one more phone call to her old college roommate, Susan, who lived in Portland with her husband Rob.

I remembered Susan as a bright, vivacious young woman who laughed easily. She had been to our home to visit when Dayna came to town. Dayna was hopeful that, somehow, there might be a chance of seeing her this time as well.

"You won't believe my timing!" Dayna, brightened by the conversation, had just hung up. "They're packing for their third trip to Africa. That's where they spent their honeymoon and they just fell in love with it. Susan said it's the most amazing place in the world. But, they'd love to meet me tomorrow if it works with our chemo schedule."

Susan and Rob lived in a beautifully maintained neighborhood in northwest Portland with charming boutiques and well-appointed homes. Coincidentally, it's also where the clinic is located, making it very convenient for Dayna to meet her friends. Although I was not sure how the chemotherapy treatment would affect me, I thought I'd be fine if she left for a while.

"Only if you're sure it's all right. The reason I'm here is you, so if I miss them, I'll just catch them next time."

"Forget it—you're going."

Monday, Rich took us to "chemo" and we assured him we'd be fine without him.

"Remember, I'm a phone call away," and he left for work.

First, the nurse took us to a room where she then attempted to access the port in my chest. She tried several times.

"This cath is built with a cup on the end that holds the drug while it infuses. Yours is at a weird angle and I can't hit the cup with the needle. This needle is supposed to go right into the center of it but it's not getting there. If I could just reach . . ."

Another nurse came to help. Normally a simple procedure, connecting me became complicated by the odd position of my shunt. I stopped counting the needle sticks when I noticed Dayna getting pale. I could tell that she was horrified.

"Annette, are you all right?"

I assured her I was fine and told the nurse to keep going.

"I know that's a lot of pokes. I'm going to give you some numbing medication. We have to keep trying until we get it." She had no choice; she had to keep sticking me.

When I looked at Dayna again, I surmised that she was worried about my fainting from the ghastly procedure.

"Oh, come on. It's not as bad as the Whipple," referring to my recent surgery. Many times in the weeks that followed I would remind myself that I made it through surgery that was much worse than anything I was now experiencing.

"It's okay, keep going."

"Let's get her a longer needle."

A four-inch needle was inserted into my chest and finally achieved its objective: it hit the cup.

Next, we were taken into the "recliner room" where I chose the seat near a window because it reminded me least of a ward. Dayna looked like she could use a walk.

"Why don't you go see Susan? I'm not going anywhere. Tell her I'm still trying to talk Rich into going to Africa, so please bring back tons of pictures. We'll see them when they get back. Besides, I have all these great books Zelda brought. Please, go. Take your time." And I tried to settle in as Dayna reluctantly left to meet her friends at a neighborhood café. She called to check on me an hour later and I convinced her to stay with them longer. This part was a piece of cake.

When Dayna returned she was very animated about Susan's trip.

"They're going to see the gorillas! It's with a tour group on a first-class expedition with guards and cooks and guides. It's really deep in the jungle and they have to set up camp in the forest, but they said it's all very safe and civilized." She told me how excited Rob was.

"They leave tomorrow and they're just so happy. Thanks for letting me sneak off with them for a while."

A few days after Dayna had gone home, she called me, sobbing. I could hardly understand her. It was about Susan and Rob. They were dead–murdered in Africa, I thought she said. But her crying was so deep that I couldn't be sure of the words. Yes, they had been abducted in the forest and murdered in Africa.

The story that unfolded described a massacre of unfathomable cruelty and sheer brutality. As a senseless and shameful political statement, a band of about 125 rebels invaded the encampment and took several prisoners. Some were tortured and murdered, Susan and Rob among them. The thoughts of their terror and suffering drove the anguish deep into Dayna's soul.

"When I think of what they did to her and how afraid she must have been . . ." She was gasping. "I just can't believe that it really happened. I'll never see her again. Oh, Annette, they're gone. Susan and Rob are gone. Their lives were so perfect and now they're gone."

I was incapable of comforting Dayna for her sorrow was impenetrable. There was nothing I could do or say to console her. All I could do was listen. As she told me the details of the news reports, the magnitude of the torment they must have endured became too vivid.

"I didn't tell you that Susan was really upset when I told her about your chemotherapy. She said she didn't know how she would handle it if she had to do it. She kept talking about how awful it must be for you. She thought she was lucky because she hadn't gotten cancer."

I had never heard her cry so deeply. She kept talking.

"I was so worried about losing you and felt really guilty about going off to see them. I was afraid I was taking precious time that you and I might be cheated out of later. If I hadn't been in Portland with you, I would have missed them, never seen them again."

The next day when I went in for treatment, I did not mind the ache in my joints or the abdominal cramps, did not feel the needle going into my chest to access my port. My task was simple compared to the story that resonated in my mind. And, as I settled into my recliner, I was struck with the realization that no one ever really knows when our time is coming.

Two weeks later, Dayna returned to Portland to stay with us while attending the memorial service for Susan and her beloved husband. The couple had worked together at Intel and had decided to splurge on one last big trip before taking a sabbatical. It was their plan to enjoy some time off together. Now, they were together forever.

11

Taking Control

True leaders emerge during times of crisis. History books are filled with victories attributed to those who make strategic decisions under extreme circumstances. What they all have in common are characteristics that cause them to act when others will not. Most approach their challenge with a methodical plan, consistently keeping their goal in focus while orchestrating the interaction of resources. First, however, they educate themselves as thoroughly as possible about their adversary.

For my entire career, it had been drilled into me that to solve a problem, I had first to understand it. As I began assessing my situation, I realized that I had relatively little scientific, factual, or useful data about my illness. My knowledge about cancer was, for the most part, a crude composition of anecdotes from friends, relatives, and celebrities. Hence, I began my basic education. Initially on the Internet, then later at the public library, I encountered an abundance of material covering everything from diagnosis to diet. There were overviews of the general nature of the disease, explaining how it invades new territory, claiming it as its own. There were detailed descriptions of specific case studies with histories, trends, and analysis. Various therapies were described including side effects, statistics, new developments, as well as alternative and homeopathic remedies. Finally, there was a mounting body of work surrounding cancer prevention. Thus, I began to gain insights into the world I was entering.

As a warning, a friend had cautioned me that the statistics could be frightening, so I should prepare myself mentally.

"As you're looking at mortality rates," she said, "remember that numbers are just numbers. The percentage of deaths could reflect patients without therapy or before new treatment was available. They could be patients of any age or with any number of complications. When you're looking at statistics, you don't really know how they apply to you. Just prepare yourself to see some difficult numbers. And, stay focused on the survivors."

It was my observation that most patients don't want granular, biological information about cancer or about the impact of treatments on the systems of the body. They simply want to be done with it. My treatments began the same way, with my being told only that which the doctors or nurses believed I needed to know. However, as I became better informed and began asking questions, my health care team was very supportive of my quest for knowledge.

Of the seven million Americans diagnosed with cancer in 1995, nearly three million were men as compared to four and a half million women. The disparity, I understood, was due to reproductive cancers. Lung cancer has the highest incidence and is three times more prevalent than the second most common cancer, colorectal. Breast cancer is third, followed by cancers of the prostate, pancreas, ovary, and leukemia.

Cancer is the second leading cause of death in the United States, exceeded only by heart disease. Cancer deaths in the United States in 1995 represented over half a million of the staggering 5.5 million cancer deaths worldwide. There are, however, greater numbers of people who are living with cancer, being treated with various combinations of surgery, radiation, chemotherapy, hormones, and immunotherapy. Over nine million Americans are living with a cancer history.

"Cancer isn't a disease but a group of diseases that are characterized by an uncontrolled growth of abnormal cells," the nurse explained while we played hide and seek with my access port. "It's the spread of these cells that can be fatal. So, treatment is essentially a strategy to stop the spread. Sometimes that means surgical removal. With other cases, we think the most effective plan is to contain the cancer and stop it from spreading. Or, as in your case, we're going for total remission, hopefully eradicating the disease once and for all."

I asked why, under similar circumstances, some people will get cancer while others don't.

"That depends on many factors, so it's not a simple answer. For example, we know that smoking can cause cancer, but why do some people smoke like a chimney and live into their nineties, while others die young from secondhand smoke? The thing is that every person's immune condition is different. In other words, how strong are your body's defenses against the carcinogens that we come in contact with every day that one person is susceptible to while another person is fortified against? Partly, it's what we inherit in our genes, but it's also how we live. Our diet can make a difference by helping the body ward off cancer or by putting us at a higher risk. You could be exposed to radiation or toxic microorganisms, even viruses, at a time when other biological factors make conditions perfect—or impossible—for cancer to grow. Or, there could be internal causes—hormones or an inherited mutation that was in your DNA but didn't fully mature into cancer until now. Unfortunately, it can be years between the cause and the effect. That's what makes it tough to draw direct correlations.

"The curious thing about ovarian cancer is that most women with the disease don't have any known risk factors. We know that granulosa cell grows from connective tissue cells around the ovary that produce estrogen and progesterone. What we don't know is why the cells become abnormal."

As I learned more about ovarian cancer, it frightened me to know that over half of the women with this illness die. In the category of women thirty-five years and older, ovarian cancer ranked fourth as the most common killer and has the highest mortality rate of all female cancers. The odds for survivors of recurrent ovarian cancer were not just pessimistic; they were dreadful.

In my quest for knowledge I found that the American Cancer Society and National Cancer Institute provided material that was clear, consistent, and succinct. The information was easily accessible on their websites and organized such that I could opt for more detail, although their information tended to be general in nature.

As I continued looking at research, I began thinking about the statistics in terms of "survival rate" versus "mortality rate." As one of my survivor friends said, "Someone makes up that four or five percent, why not me?"

Yes, why not me?

The treatments began their work and, in doing so, produced a series of physical and emotional challenges for which I was unprepared. It is impossible to imagine without having personally experienced it and it differs for each person and for each therapy. For me, it was not the actual chemotherapy infusions that were uncomfortable. In truth, once my port was accessed and I was "connected," there was no physical sensation at all. It was the side effects—the nausea, fatigue, and cramps that made me ill. Additionally, some of the adjunct treatments, such as shots, compounded the problem with their own set of symptoms, like aching in my joints.

I was also afraid. There were many different kinds of fear and they were all paramount in my mind. I was afraid of the actual experience I was going through, as though fighting a battle that was completely unknown to me, making me unsure of myself. Also, I was frightened of the effects of chemotherapy drugs on my body. Ultimately, I was afraid that the therapy would not save my life.

It was exactly two and a half weeks into treatment that my hair fell out. For some reason I had expected a gradual loss. Then, one day as I was shampooing it, I lathered up the mass of hair and was shocked to find my hands full of dead hair. It looked like I was holding a wig. I expected it, knew it was coming, but still I wept. Chemotherapy had killed the hair roots and left a reminder of what was once full, thick, chocolate brown hair.

William shaved my head as I watched in the mirror.

"Are you all right?"

"Oh, sure. It's only hair." My tears flowed with a mind of their own.

For the first time I saw how sick I looked. Being without hair made me look pitiful and that made me terribly sad. I had entered the world of chemotherapy with great reluctance. I resisted identifying with the other patients and still did not regard myself as one of them. Generally, I kept to myself. What I had in common with the others was something I wished I didn't have at all, a potentially fatal disease. Now I had crossed the border into their world. I had become one of them.

Then one day, I was approached by a beautiful woman who was being treated for breast cancer for the second time. I was glad when our schedules for infusions overlapped because she always seemed to have a positive, upbeat attitude about her. She asked how I was doing with it all, sensing my misery. I told her how upset I was about losing my hair and yet feeling confused by my reaction. It seemed to be a bit irrational since losing my hair was the one thing that would hurt the least and it would come back most easily. Yet the event had shaken me emotionally. It seemed to be one more insult heaped on top of all the indignities I had already suffered, I told her, and it upset me that now my condition was no longer private. Not now, with my bald head as evidence to the world that I was an official member of the Chemo Club.

She smiled and told me her story.

"Since this is a repeat for me, well, my husband knew what to expect. He knew I would be pretty upset 'cause I was last time. When it looked like my hair was starting to go, you know how you see a lot of hair on your pillow or in the shower? Well, he planned this wonderful dinner for just the two of us. He cooked everything himself. He had candles and wine and our good china. It was real romantic. Well, after dinner he ceremoniously shaved my head himself and then, he made love to me." She smiled with a love that I knew she carried deep inside, in a place where the chemicals cannot go.

The chemotherapy nurses at the treatment center were a surprise to me. I had a plethora of nurse experiences, most of them positive. I expected a competent group of nurses who would administer treatments the same way the nurse in the doctor's office takes blood, efficient but impersonal. What I found instead was a very compassionate team, concerned about each of us as individuals. They knew every patient's personal situation and empathized with each one. They remembered the conversation you had with them yesterday and what your husband or wife looked like and whether or not you liked being by the window. And, their main concern, beyond the necessary infusions, was the comfort of their patients. They would try anything in their arsenal of drugs to reduce the side effects. By the second cycle, I had dispatched my Ghost of Cancers Past and was able to see the logic of treatments in the "recliner room." This wasn't a terminal cancer ward in Houston from my childhood. It was a clean operation with efficient procedures, caring personnel, and the best developments of modern medicine. Still, I was slow to open up to the others who shared this facility and this fight with me.

When I first became ill, I was reluctant to complain about my condition. It was not in my nature to do so. I was hesitant to bother the twenty-four-hour medical service unless it was a full-fledged emergency, thinking that, if I was feeling bad, I should just "tough it out." I was told to expect "flu-like symptoms" from injections meant to restore my blood cells. Shortly after one round of shots, I was hit with extreme pain that made me feel more like a victim of a motorcycle accident. I lay in bed wondering how I could repeat this ten days in a row. Then, luckily, one of my chemo friends called to check on me. As I described my physical indications, she told me to hang up and call the nurse because what I was feeling wasn't right. Once I called in, I found that I was having an allergic reaction to a shot and had suffered for hours unnecessarily. The nurse from the service insisted that they were available for general questions as well as specific problems and that this was a service for me to use at my discretion.

Generally, I became better at communicating; comparing notes with other patients to learn what was helping them. I questioned procedures to learn how and why they worked. For every major decision, I asked my doctors for a clear understanding of the worst and best possible outcomes, knowing that if my probing was unwelcome, I should change doctors.

"Time to go to work," Rich would chirp, a bounce in his step as he started every day. He acted like our lives were perfectly ordinary and we were simply commuting to work together. Every day, he would help me get ready and off we would go. He referred to my treatments as my "job." We all had our jobs to do.

"Bye, honey. Have a good day at work. I'll try to come by at noon," as he dropped me off at the treatment center, a big smile on his face. Although I appreciated his positive attitude, at times I envied his optimism.

"Sometimes I feel defeated," I confided in Dennis, "like I don't know what I did to deserve this."

Dennis knew that as things got tougher, it would be critical to stay committed to the substantial physical and psychological demands of my treatments.

"This isn't a punishment or a reward. You know it doesn't work that way. Besides, this condition might have been dialed into your genes generations ago. Who knows? The important thing now is not *why* you have it, but rather, *what* you intend to do about it. It doesn't mean you shouldn't be angry or sad that this has occurred in your life. Have the feelings, wholly and completely. I would be concerned if you didn't have them. Have them. Then I want you to let them go. They usurp energy that you can't afford to give up right now. You have to have control."

With practice I was learning to vent my raw emotions, then compartmentalize them and "just put them away." This freed me to concentrate on what I intended to do about what was happening to me.

"For you to be the person you are today you made tough choices and then you acted on them. Something within you, some inner voice caused you to change the facts that surrounded your life. Think back to those times and tell me what you see."

To my mind's eye was lifted a kaleidoscope of memories, each piece individually distinct yet part of a bigger pattern, interlocked rather than integrated. The images moved between and among each other, reminding me vividly of events long retired. These glimpses of my past revealed the conditioning that had taken place over a lifetime of dealing with life's problems and prospects. A child whose daily objective was to escape danger became a defiant young woman who could face her fears.

"As soon as I was able, I changed my life . . . first in little ways, breaking away from the well-worn path, then more ambitiously as I gained confidence and skill and opportunity."

The first major turning point in my adult life occurred when I moved away from Texas. In 1972, at age twenty-two, I drove from Texas to Washington, D.C. to start a new life. During the next five years, I would change everything about myself.

Switching from liberal arts to a business track, I began taking classes at night while working in customer service for business accounts. As I began the rapid assimilation into a complex world of commerce that had been unknown to me, I found that my interest in and ability to learn business came easily. I became intrigued by the logic of it and began thinking in systematic terms about life in general.

For me, living in Washington was exhilarating. Politically, it was an exciting time. Nixon was in office and we began hearing rumors of a cover-up. Then, Watergate. It was sensational. History was being made and I was seeing it unfold all around me.

There were many other benefits to my new home, such as a phenomenal choice of political and cultural events. World experts routinely gave free lectures and performing arts were available to suit anyone's taste. At trendy bars on the Hill, staffers exposed the gritty side of politics while, next door, extravagant international affairs were being staged by the diplomatic sector. I studied the people as well as the issues, learning everything that I could absorb. Growing up as I did, with no prior exposure to refinement, I now lived in the only city in America that still used finger bowls.

It was during this time that my first adult friendship was formed. It was the early seventies when, as a result of a federal government mandate, industry was forced to open its "male-only" jobs to women. My subsequent promotion into a sales position resulted in my being the first woman in my new group. For me it was awkward and intimidating in that not all workers embraced the change. At the time there was a dearth of female role models and I was perplexed as to how to gain acceptance. So it was that a senior sales executive named Walter became my first mentor.

"If they seem hostile, it's because you represent change," he spoke with wisdom beyond his years. "Most people aren't comfortable with change, especially when it's forced on them. But, it's not personal—so don't take it personally. Just show them. Perform at your best." Hence, the coaching began.

Whether confused by the group dynamics, the foreign culture, or the intense corporate politics, I knew that I could go to Walter for counsel. Recognizing that I had an aptitude for business, he took me under his wing and gave me safe harbor in the unfamiliar and often stormy waters.

"Create an honest balance between 'fitting in' and being yourself. Never forget that you live with Annette more than you live with them."

By peeling back layer after layer, he exposed the strengths and weaknesses of decisions and decision makers. He demystified the upper echelon of management, enabling me to aspire to greater advancement.

Walter, with Gloria, his wife, also had a profound impact on my personal style. Originally from New England, they now made their home in the historic community of Manassas, Virginia. They became my surrogate family, inviting me for holiday meals and Sunday dinner. Enchanted by the Victorian passion for grandeur, Gloria unveiled the distinctive style of Washington formality and etiquette, while Walter taught me the value of handcrafted objects that showed the pride of the maker in the carving of a cabinet or its hand-forged hinge.

"Do you realize that these pieces have held up for over a hundred years? Look at their beauty, the strength, and the character. What could we possibly make today that someone will cherish a hundred years from now?" He said it always with respect, but tinged with a touch of regret.

After five years enjoying single life in the nation's capital, I was ready for a new challenge. The west coast beckoned, with its flash and cash, the nucleus of a computer revolution. I transferred to the Santa Clara Valley in time to replace an incompetent person who had mangled a critical military communications upgrade for our most prestigious customer. The problem had been hidden from management by my predecessor and was now impacting the customer's mission by delaying satellite launches at the cost of hundreds of millions of dollars to the military and its stable of contractors. It took weeks to unravel the mess but once done, the project was completed on time and the risk to the company was mitigated. With my credibility firmly established, I was on my way.

I told Dennis of numerous examples of successful pursuits, things that women from my background did not normally do, such as climbing the ladder through the ranks, reaching senior management after a dozen promotions. At the time of my illness, I was enjoying an accomplished career at USWEST, developing business at the high end of the company's markets since 1990. My work in education and rural health care technology positioned me as a spokesperson at the national policy level, allowing me to influence political agendas that impacted millions of people.

A Hispanic woman holding executive appointments at that time was an extraordinary feat in American industry, a unique opportunity that allowed me to use my position as a platform for change. Advocacy for women and minorities became a crusade, fueled by the prospect of bringing enlightenment to corporate diversity policies.

As Dennis and I examined the steps I had taken to redirect my life, I came to the realization that during my struggle over the last few months I had lost my sense of identity. Nothing in my new existence was familiar, nothing normal. Therefore, the normal reactions I would have to adversarial situations were not engaged.

"Mentally and spiritually, you should have a feeling of moving yourself toward wellness. Do you remember Viktor Frankl, the Austrian Jew who was imprisoned by the Nazis? He talks about people overcoming incredible conditions because they had the will to live. There are many examples where a man's desire to be healed was the greatest factor contributing to his survival. This can be as powerful a force as your medications, if not more so. We need to develop a mindset that says 'this is what I do to get well so that I can reach my life goal.' In essence, it is what you have been doing intuitively all of your life. Let's shift your thinking to that of your will to live."

I recalled recovering from cancer the first time and questioning my life choices, wondering how to get it right and finally figuring it out. I began working with Dennis to anchor my vision.

"So, what is different about your marriage to Rich?"

"I married Rich because I cannot imagine not being married to him. I have to live my life with this man and him with me. I never had to think about it. Being married to him is not about something else, like getting me to a certain place. Being married to Rich is all about being married to Rich. Our relationship is what we do. We have a huge variety of activities we're involved in but they are always in support of our relationship."

"Is that why you two never fight?" Dennis remembered.

"Precisely. It's like arguing with yourself. What's the point? Instead, we tend to look at situations like we're two sides of one brain. Reasoning things through with Rich is gratifying and stimulating. One of the great things about him is his perspective on life: he sees the world as it should be and just tries to put things right when they're out of order.

"I believe that my greatest accomplishment in life is being capable of loving and being loved so completely. Rich and I have absolute love. Absolute love means absolute vulnerability, and absolute vulnerability means absolute trust. It's the best feeling in the world."

I knew then that I was not afraid to die; I was simply not ready to stop living. A will to live? Yes, I had a will to live. Before this, my life was truly fulfilled and I wanted it back. I had a tremendous will to live.

In trance, I heard Dennis say, "You are not a sick person. You are a healthy person having a traumatic experience," his voice anchoring the thoughts in my subconscious mind. "Your mind is healthy and your spirit is strong. You are surrounded by intense love. These things have caused you to make a choice to live. It dictates the way you process every thought that passes through your brain, consciously and subconsciously," he said, weaving a web of psychological and spiritual reinforcement.

"What does wellness look like to you? Paint the picture for me." He spoke as though it were a place on a map, "Wellnessville," with avenues and trees.

I had felt it and sensed it but had not described it in that way.

"Wellness? Well it's no pain and no pills. It's Rich taking the children out on the boat on a sunny day, me sitting beside him holding a grandbaby." There were thousands of versions of my response, all continuations of the great love in our life.

"It's seeing the latest movie with Rich and sitting together," I laughed. Before I became ill, we went to the movies every Friday night. But when my sense of smell changed, one smell that repulsed me was that of popcorn. This presented a problem for Rich because he is incapable of watching the big screen without it. That meant he couldn't sit near me until he'd finish his bag. Wellness meant going again, but this time, we'd sit together.

Wellness was no longer puking every day. Sitting in a restaurant enjoying a meal with my friends. Shopping without people pretending not to see. Sleeping six or seven hours straight through the night.

Wellness was also me in my professional role, making decisions, arguing causes, running with the ball. My corporate identity was a huge part of who I was.

By this point in my life, I had developed a habit of winning. For years, I had been making the daily decisions required to lead groups of people during turbulent times. Trained at top management colleges to use tools and targets to quantify and qualify progress, I had taken charge of numerous multimillion-dollar projects, successfully delivering results within strict technical and cost guidelines. World-class experts in the field of systematic process management had honed my ability to use scientific methods, removing subjectivity in order to arrive at solutions that were logical and rational and real. Yet, now facing the most important project of my life, I realized that I had no winning game plan.

Drawing on skills from my professional development, I decided to approach my problem strategically, to come at it from every possible angle in order to create the highest possible probability for success. As I formulated what would have to be done, the solution began to take on the shape of a managed project.

As I looked around my universe, I realized that I was surrounded by an abundance of resources with a broad range of competencies and untapped potential. I was not alone; I had a ferocious support system. Beyond my doctors and nurses, family and friends, there were avenues of support that I had not yet considered, a vast network of knowledge and skill waiting to be discovered.

Now, I was able to focus on my situation more objectively. My training demanded that I set my feelings aside in order to examine my problem scientifically. What levers could be pulled to impact my situation? What variables should we track and why? How could we get regular, meaningful measurements? I began thinking about quantitative data, things that were factual and measurable, such as lab reports. Next, the data would have to be relevant, like body composition readings that measure lean muscle mass gains and losses. We dealt with subjective indicators, such as how I was feeling, by assigning a value or number that we could compare. For example, on a scale of one to ten, how nauseous was I today? Or, if yesterday's pain level had been a seven, would today be an eight or a six?

My daily obsession became the successful alleviation of my illness and a return to health. I experienced a shift in my attention, contemplating the outcome of my treatment rather than dwelling on the agony of it. From the time of my admission to the hospital, I had lived with the thought of dying. At some point I cannot remember, the thought had dissipated like the morning dew, unnoticed and unmissed.

Joanne had a benchmark for my body composition, muscular strength, aerobic fitness, and general physical condition from shortly before I became ill. Now, she used a skin-fold caliper to assess my body's muscle/fat content in order to track the changes during chemotherapy. Her findings alarmed her. I had now lost fifty-five pounds in two months, over half of which was muscle. We knew that if we did not stop the loss of muscle mass, my recovery would be even harder.

During this time I felt terrible. I was tired all the time and every action was an effort. Muscle atrophy had set in rapidly in the hospital and my legs and buttocks were uncharacteristically skinny. The chemotherapy side effects picked up where the surgery left off, attacking my whole body, from faulty cognition to nausea and vomiting, fatigue, diarrhea, and anorexia. I was weak and getting weaker, and I was still losing weight.

It wasn't that I was "just not hungry," I couldn't eat at all. The mere thought of some foods made me ill. Sweets tasted a thousand times sweeter and some foods I had loved, like chocolate, now had a disgusting aroma. Cooking, one of my favorite pastimes, was now repugnant.

"I'm worried about you." It was Joanne, of course. Everyone else told me how great I looked. Not Joanne—she was always truthful.

"If you lose all your muscle strength now, how are you going to go through recovery? I'm not just talking about how you manage chemotherapy. I'm talking about fighting infections and regenerating new tissue and saving your skin and teeth and bones. I know you're trying but I'm very concerned about how you will emerge from this experience."

Joanne was questioning my ability to bear up under the long, difficult therapy. She proposed the idea of approaching food differently—from the standpoint of supporting the body's needs at this particular time. It was easier to understand once she taught us the principles involved.

"Metabolism is the process of turning food into energy that can be used by the body to perform all the things it has to do. Naturally, we tend to think of needing energy for voluntary activities, like walking or talking or exercising—all the stuff we choose to do. Actually, the voluntary part accounts for only 35 or 40 percent of your energy requirements. The other 55 to 60 percent is what the body needs to fuel its involuntary functions—your circulation and respiration, creating heat to maintain your body temperature, all your nerve activity, and synthesizing new tissue and secreting hormones and on and on. Every function of your body, every system, every particle requires energy. That's what we call 'basal metabolism,' as in base or fundamental: the metabolism necessary to just be alive.

"If we take a woman who weighs an average one hundred twenty pounds whose basal metabolic rate is roughly 1600 calories and add another 860 calories for voluntary activity, we get a total of 2460 calories—under normal conditions. The catch is that both illness and stress raise the basal metabolic rate, meaning that you need even more calories to repair your body after surgery, to fight infection and build new blood and tissue, and to manage anxiety or tension. Then, add chemotherapy on top of that and I can't even calculate your body's demands right now."

I knew I wasn't eating enough to reach the conservative estimate of my body's needs. Some foods moved through me so rapidly that it seemed useless to eat anything. On the other hand, I very much wanted to know how to feel better, not worse. If my goal was to create the best possible outcome to my situation, my actions were not supporting it. I needed a specific plan, one that would give me a nutritionally sound foundation to support all the systems of my body.

The diet was devised with a dual focus on quantity (calories) and quality (food groups). Beyond assuring that I consumed enough calories, Joanne introduced the combination of foods that she believed provided the optimum nutrients for energy, repair, and rebuilding of my immune function. She stressed that this approach was well studied by nutritionists and was considered the essential underpinning to the restoration of my health.

The diet was based on the American Cancer Society recommendations, with a food balance in the following proportions:

*Carbohydrates - at least 55%, from grains, starches, fruits, vegetables, legumes.
*Protein - preferably 25%, but at least 15%, from fish, meat, grains, legumes, dairy, eggs, soy.
*Fat - limited to 20%

I remembered that proteins were considered the "building blocks" for new cells and wondered why protein represented only one-fourth of the foods on the diet. Wouldn't a high protein diet be better?

"Carbohydrates are the most readily available food source which makes them the main fuel supply," Joanne explained. "It's because they're easier for the body to break down and use. Your body resorts to consuming lean muscle because if no other food source is available, it has to choose from what's left. Losing muscle is less important than losing organs, so your body is really designed to work that way when it is in a state of starvation. The problem is that this compounds your fatigue, making you even less active, causing you to lose even more muscle.

"Believe me, if you're eating enough, twenty-five percent from proteins will cover your needs."

Why fat?

"Fat shouldn't be eliminated because you need it to metabolize vitamins and nutrients. It's also essential for smooth and healthy skin, hair, and nails, which are all being hit pretty hard by the therapy. Of course, too much fat can limit your body's efficiency at repairing itself, so you really need to monitor it. If you need extra calories, it's really best to get them from carbs."

With that, we applied Joanne's guidelines to the daily planning of each meal. The problem for us was measuring, since only a portion of what I ingested would reach its destination due to increased vomiting and the hyper-motility from surgery. This meant that eating more food, not less, was critical.

Initially, we customized a diet that concentrated on the following foods:

Fish, chicken, and pork were boiled, broiled, baked, or sautéed in olive oil.

Vegetables and fruits were peeled, cooked, juiced, or blended.

Eggs were prepared in any way I could tolerate them.

Dairy, organic if possible, was introduced in snacks of cheese or yogurt.

Soy, in a variety of forms, was used as a dairy substitute.

Grains from breads, tortillas, crackers, rice, and pasta were easier to digest.

Potatoes, "the food of last resort," were as reliable as any food could be. When all else fails, eat mashed potatoes. With instant potatoes, I could fix them myself.

Legumes included peanut butter, hummus, and beans.

Liquid supplements added balanced nutrients between meals.

Fluids included at least two liters of water per day, to counteract vomiting, dehydration, and to flush the chemicals through my system.

And, in response to recent cancer prevention and treatment

alternatives, we added foods found to have beneficial properties, such as green tea, soy, avocado, and fish oil.

We sometimes used bland foods as a vehicle to get other higher-value foods to stay down; for example, potatoes or pasta were useful for adding cheese, meat, or beans to the diet. Sushi was the only food I craved and was miraculously well tolerated. Soups were best at night because they were less uncomfortable if they came back up. Greasy foods were not at all tolerable. Bile is needed to emulsify fat, causing more acid to enter the stomach, resulting in more violent vomiting.

We avoided processed meats, carbonated drinks, highly acidic or hard-to-digest foods, alcoholic beverages, and food with no nutritional value. Variety was important because some foods worked when others didn't. At times foods differed by the way they were prepared, so we got creative and experimented. It was trial and error on a daily basis. For example, eggs could go either way—great one day but the next, forget about it.

Tracy and William observed that my ability to think seemed impaired at times. I had been exhibiting symptoms of forgetfulness, confusion, loss of words, or entire events. I believed that I could reason with near-normal accuracy but, simultaneously, could not remember what day comes after Wednesday. I could no longer rely on my memory about the day's consumption; I had to write it down.

William started to overlay the schedule of daily feedings with medications and procedures, creating a master chart. Now, our thoughts about food shifted to my need to create fuel.

"From now on," Tracy announced one day, "we'll just get meals in front of you at the appointed time, you eat what you can, and we'll try and measure it." At times, she would resort to tactics she used with her toddler. "Do you want the peanut butter or the cheese sandwich?"

We also discovered that my nausea was worse at night, which I attributed to my lying in bed while dead cells built up in the stomach, provoking another attack. To deal with this, we adjusted my meals to load most of the calories into the middle of the day, thus improving my chances for nourishment.

We kept track of the foods and times and results, not in an absolutely mechanical way but with an awareness every day about volume, balance, and outcome. We had enough information to help us make decisions. For instance, the log told us that I consumed and retained more when eating frequent small meals rather than having breakfast, lunch, and dinner. I was given something to eat every two hours from then on.

In summary, the diet was designed with a dual purpose: first, to generate sufficient fuel to sustain my body's functions without having to devour its stored resources; and to support my body's ability to rebuild and restore itself. My diet was customized to my condition and tastes, and it represented foods available to me. Also, it represented a goal or guideline for daily consumption, even though there were many days when my actual consumption fell short.

A sample of the diet is presented here for illustrative purposes. Any diet should be designed specifically to one's condition and tastes. This diet may not be effective or appropriate for others, although it was of tremendous benefit to me.

Sample Daily Diet

7:00	Breakfast: egg scrambled with cream, 1 slice toast, butter, tea or juice.
9:00	Snack: 1 oz cheese and 4 crackers, or 4 oz yogurt
Noon	Lunch: 2 oz roasted chicken breast, 1/4 cup cooked vegetables
2:00	Snack: 2 oz cheese, bread, or fruit
4:00	Snack: 6 oz liquid protein supplement
6:00	Dinner: 4 oz fish, 1/4 cup potatoes, and 1/4 cup vegetables
8:00	Snack: protein-rich liquid supplement

In addition to improved nutrition, we evolved in other ways as well. We had begun thinking as a team, approaching my cancer with control mechanisms according to a plan designed to improve my condition. We became organized and made decisions, working together to identify problems and analyze them in practical ways.

Dr. Tseng was impressed by my tolerance for the treatments. I was holding up well, better than most women following my protocol of therapy. His feedback was encouraging and the team was proud of our progress. Best of all, the plan was working.

Todd Siler, whom I thanked repeatedly for getting me to journal, remained closely connected during this time. Through research associates at M.I.T. he had discovered information on experimental life extension protocols for cancer patients. The work concluded that certain nutrition regimens used in support of oncology have been found to reduce the toxicity of the drug therapy.

"The underlying premise of this work is that cancer is not just limited to the tumor but is a disease that involves the entire body." He sent us the research, then he called to explain that there were three main conclusions that we needed to know about.

"First you have to remember that the body is engineered to protect itself. It has certain triggers that cause different biological events to occur. If you use nutrition as a complementary therapy to engage those triggers, you can increase the odds of your remission. In other words, use the entire body to fight." He spoke of an ecosystem.

"Next, nutrition can make chemotherapy and radiation more selectively toxic to the cancer cells. And, of course, nutrition therapy stimulates your immune function and minimizes malnutrition."

The material he showed us professed compelling results with a reasonable diet of unprocessed food low in fat, dairy, and sugar, coupled with therapeutic doses of vitamins and minerals, *in conjunction with conventional oncology care*. The trials, sponsored by the National Cancer Institute, recommended nutrition therapy to improve the conditions of the body that discourage the growth of cancer cells by using certain foods and vitamins with cancer-fighting properties, such as avocado, green tea, whey protein, and garlic. We read that soy protein containing several anti-cancer agents may lower the prevalence of prostate cancer and inhibit estrogen-positive human breast cancer cells. The only caution was for patients with estrogen-receptor-positive breast cancer.

"Look at what happened with lung patients." Todd, excited at the finding, wondered why it was not common knowledge that lung patients who consumed more vegetables lived significantly longer.

"If changes in diet could significantly increase their life span beyond the normal expectations, why don't the 150,000 Americans with lung cancer know this?"

Then there were the vitamins. The report stated that Vitamin A inhibits cancer cell proliferation, particularly in cancer of the mouth. Vitamin D, also thought to inhibit cancer cell growth, is being studied as a way to change prostate cancer and breast cancer cells back to normal under laboratory conditions. Studies were being conducted to test fish oil in reducing pancreatic cancer cells and inhibiting metastasis of breast and lung cancer. Vitamin C is listed because of its antioxidant content. Echinacea, popular because of its ability to boost the immune system, was found to have profound anti-cancer effects in patients suffering from metastasized cancers of the colon and esophagus.

Melatonin, which I had taken for insomnia, "boosts immune system function, suppresses free radicals, inhibits cell proliferation, and helps to change cancer cells back to normal cells." (The study discouraged its use by patients with leukemia, Hodgkin's disease, and lymphoma.)

All of the studies stressed that "they should not be used by themselves in case of illness" and were intended as supportive nutritional information for patients and their physicians, with specific dosages determined individually in consultation with a health care professional.

Organic fruits and vegetables, organic dairy and eggs, and fish were also recommended. Some foods considered high-risk were discouraged, such as foods that are processed, hormone-laden meat and dairy products, and any foods with additives or chemical processing.

We shifted my diet to concentrate on fish and vegetables with rice, potatoes, or noodles. We tried to buy organic produce, dairy, and eggs, but the costs for some were still unreasonable and often we compromised. Also, we added soy products and green tea whenever possible.

"It says here that the group with the lowest incidence of cancer is Chinese women who drink about ten cups of green tea a day." We stepped up the green tea. After all, I wasn't drinking coffee or sodas.

Every day Rich and I went through our little breakfast ritual.

"I scrambled you some eggs, made some toast and here's juice. Just stay in bed a few more minutes; I'll bring it to you." He would pretend he hadn't heard me retching all night and climbed the stairs to our bedroom with a tray of food. Every day he made me breakfast, and almost every day, I threw it up. After a while, it didn't bother us because for us, it was normal.

I had no idea what it would be like to be nauseous day after day, for months at a time. As my treatment progressed, my vomiting became more severe until it reached a point where, some days and most nights, it was virtually nonstop. I would sometimes sleep standing by the lavatory, my head resting on a towel between episodes. I worried about disturbing Rich night after night because the nausea was worsening. I was now fatigued most of the time, but on especially bad days, I was completely exhausted. Also, constant vomiting was particularly painful considering that my surgeries involved all the major abdominal organs.

"Have you tried marijuana?" asked one of my veteran friends. "It worked for me."

At this point I would try anything. The pills weren't cutting it anymore and I was losing weight again. Worried about pulmonary setbacks, I decided to check with the lung specialist and with my nurses, neither of which was concerned since the usage was for a limited time.

"Isn't it legal for medicinal purposes in Oregon?" I had recently voted in support of the new law, thinking it cruel to deny cancer patients any form of effective relief.

"Yes, but it's taking a long time for the regulators to respond to requests because it's too new. They don't have it all figured out yet, like where you buy the government's product. By the time you get through the process, you could be at the end of your treatment. You might be better off finding your own source." Clearly, the nurse had been asked this before.

It did work, not by inducing the euphoric state one normally associates with being high, but rather a detachment from the discomfort of being nauseous. One major cause of the nausea is the sloughing-off of the cells that line the stomach. This happens because anti-cancer drugs kill all fast-growing cells, including those that line the esophagus and the stomach. The effect is involuntary regurgitation in an effort to expel the dead cells. The marijuana diminished the feeling of constantly needing to throw up. It also added some appetite and softened the post-operative abdominal pain.

There were times when nothing was effective because the treatments were creating a buildup of toxins. It was an ongoing battle to mitigate the effects of the harsh therapies that began to show on my face, pale, with no eyebrows, sunken and sad. I was gaunt and sleep-deprived, and I avoided looking at the spent woman in the mirror. But Rich would not have it. He came home with gifts like scarves and flowers. He would flirt or tease at unexpected times, reassuring me when I needed it.

Nearly every weekend Rich took me to the hospital for hydration, infusions of fluid with supplements of whatever I was missing. The bags of fluid were refrigerated until I arrived so the infusions felt as though ice chips were being shot into my veins. This would last up to three hours, both Saturday and Sunday. At times, I was given a heating pad to offset the cold but it was only marginally effective because of the extreme cold flowing through my veins, chilling me from the inside out.

It was one Sunday in March when the winter stubbornly refused to release its hold on the Pacific Northwest. It was then, after one of these sessions, that I simply could not shake the cold.

"Annette, come sit by the fire. I'll make some hot tea."

We had just gotten home from the hospital and Rich was my nurse now. He brought a huge, green knitted comforter, a wonderful get-well gift from a friend. He bolstered the layers of clothing I was wearing, trying heavier socks, a warmer scarf on my bald head, anything that might cut through the cold.

"I'm still freezing."

I felt ice run in my veins, carried to every place my blood flowed.

I was committed to being up every day, even if only to sit in a chair or on the sofa. We had agreed that I should resist the temptation to go to bed during the day, unless specifically for a nap. But that Sunday, I didn't care about rules. The chill was becoming an ache now, my joints picking up the discomfort and joining the complaint. All I wanted was to get warm.

"Can you get the heater going upstairs? I think I need to go to bed." I was quivering and my lips felt like they were blue.

I could tell that Rich was worried as he walked me upstairs, not sure exactly what to do for me. He covered me with quilts and turned up the heater, yet I continued to shiver, as frigid as though I lay under a blanket of snow. I then felt him climb into bed with me, rubbing my arms quickly to generate warmth, embracing me, passing his body's higher temperature on to me. I could feel the heat radiating out of him, melting the crystalline cells that I thought had surely begun to form in my blood. I felt soothed and my own warmth began to be restored. At last, I felt my body relax. Rich held me tight and held me close until I stopped shaking. Then, like embers forgotten, my own heat became kindled and soon desire was washing away the pain. I knew this place where he was taking me, knew that I was safe and protected there. I was enveloped in the love I have for this man and the sensual responses that it ignited. It did not matter that I was bald or pale or physically scarred. It did not matter what happened yesterday or what might happen tomorrow. We touched and felt and loved as any healthy, happy couple, giving pleasure to each other and to our-

selves, naturally and beautifully and completely in the moment.
And I was warm.

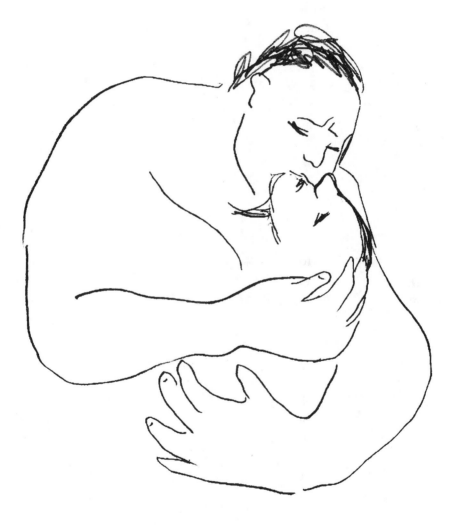

12

Friends Are Powerful Medicine

In the middle of April, the girlfriends planned another visit. I began calling us the "Ya Yas," referring to the book by Rebecca Wells about funny, spirited women in a lifetime friendship, *Divine Secrets of the Ya-Ya Sisterhood*.

Shirley arrived first and sat with us at the kitchen table. Rich asked about her husband and two teenage daughters.

"Well, they're sick as dogs. It's this winter flu and they keep it passing back and forth. It feels like they've had it all season. They just can't seem to get rid of it."

"Gee, I've been lucky this season," the words spilling out before I thought about them. "I haven't even had a cold."

Rich and Shirley were frozen, looking at each other, the preposterous statement I had made still hanging in the air. Suddenly, we all laughed and laughed and laughed. We laughed harder than we had in months.

"You nearly died in the hospital. Now, you're poisoning yourself to get rid of cancer. But, thank God, you don't have a cold!" No match for Shirley's sharp wit in my condition, I was still counting my good fortune. I actually had begun to think of myself as lucky.

The next day, Zelda arrived and was genuinely excited by my

sanguine spirits and reasonable physical condition. We made Rich listen to war stories over sushi again and for a couple of hours we were just having fun, on break from the emotional and physical strain. After dinner, Shirley, Zelda, and I sat in our guest room, as though it were a college dorm, catching up on a thousand things important only to friends. Still in my wig, I talked to them about the loss of my hair.

"So do you want to see?" And the women from whom I held no secrets now looked on as I removed the fake hair that masked my naked illness.

They were shaken more than I thought they would be, struck by the obvious damage to my body. Later, both told me of their struggle to control their reactions until I left the room, and only when in privacy, crying for me. But, it was why they were here; they had come because true friends share all things.

Dayna arrived the next day and together they threw a birthday party for Rich, knowing that it would make me happiest of all. We sang and played and laughed late into the night until Rich surrendered and went to bed while I fought the sleep, refusing to waste any of our precious time together.

As I studied these women, I was struck by the quality of humankind surrounding me. They exemplified character of the highest caliber, with depth and intelligence and selfless generosity. These were friends, not merely of the heart or mind, but friends of the soul. I was genuinely amazed to be among them.

Starting that weekend, we decided that our plan needed to set aside time to laugh and be happy. Also, we avoided sad situations or events, not simply to give ourselves time away from the agony, but rather to ameliorate the depression, which itself has been shown to hinder the body's immune system.

Many people came to offer support, but a recurring theme emerged from them: unless they had been through it themselves, most didn't know what would be okay. Knowing that their concern was genuine, we helped our friends be friends. We began thinking of them as part of our resource pool, and we suggested ways they could help that were useful to us, such as picking up a prescription or groceries or taking me shopping for a hat.

Once, a golf partner of Rich's was diagnosed with colon cancer and was undergoing exhaustive radiation and chemotherapy treatments. Rich and some of their buddies invited their friend to ride around in a golf cart while they played a round of golf. It was a barrel of laughs on a beautiful day. Although an unlikely pastime for a critically ill patient, they all had a great time.

This illness means months of daily treatments surrounded by sick strangers. Contact with my healthy friends reassured me and tethered me to my normal world. It kept me linked to the things I cared about before the illness and would care about again afterward. Those who were involved during my illness bonded to us the special way that comes of sharing one of the most intimate of life's experiences.

There were, however, some people we had thought of as close friends who surprised us with their silence. We heard from more than one that they were unsure if I wanted people to see me in my condition, yet the last thing I wanted was to feel isolated or quarantined. As I pondered this, I thought back to times when I should have been a better friend but had not known what to do and ultimately did nothing. I felt ashamed for my ignorance.

"But I thought of us as good friends. We've worked on the same team for several years." I voiced my puzzlement during my sessions with Dennis. "My feelings are hurt."

"You can only know your reality, not someone else's. You can't know what is happening in someone else's head. Maybe they don't know what to do. They may care but feel helpless themselves. Or, the situation may drag up painful memories for them about a loss they experienced at some time. The fact is, you don't really know, do you?"

"No."

"So what? So, what does it have to do with your plan?"

"Nothing."

"Maybe you should think about letting go of things that won't help you right now, like your assumptions about other people's motivations." Cut to the bone.

Under hypnosis, I pictured myself writing my assumptions, one by one, on imaginary, little pieces of white paper, then, letting each one go until they had all fluttered away. Gone. And what came into focus was the abundance of love that surrounded me.

A faithful friend is the medicine of life.
Ecclesiastes 6:16

13

Rebuilding

My physical changes during cancer therapy can be categorized in three stages: wasting, rebuilding, and recovery. By changing my diet and increasing physical activity, we began stemming the tide of muscle deterioration; we were no longer losing ground. However, my level of fatigue kept me from exercising enough to rebuild new muscle.

By the last part of therapy the drugs had evidently built up in my system and it became more painful to keep moving. The shots administered during my "off" week produced a feeling like hot lead pouring into my joints and slowly turning my bones to metal. There were many days when I wished I could sleep through the day so that it was one less day I would have to endure the misery. For me it was a new feeling, that feeling of waking up blue, dark blue. It made my skin very heavy, too heavy to get up. The temptation to stay in bed was tremendous.

The last five years of my life with Rich had been the happiest I could imagine. I reasoned that I could endure anything if it meant that I could have another five years. It was undeniably a sweet deal: day by day, I was trading one day of treatment for five more years. It became my daily obsession: five more years with Rich. With that, I got up every day, and, once I was moving, the blue blanket usually fell away.

Years ago, a mentor shared his key to success in the corporate world. "Draw bigger circles," he had coached. "When you're faced with a very difficult problem, share it with others who could potentially help you. You know, draw them into your circle. Get people interested in your problem and you'll be surprised at how invested they'll be in finding a solution."

During my career, I had become skilled at bringing talented people into projects I was responsible for and engaging them to help in accomplishing my mission. By applying the same approach to my recovery, I found that it also worked with personal issues. In the beginning, there were times when William could not leave me to go fill a prescription and it meant we paid for medications to be delivered. Later, as I got stronger and less dependent on William, I found that there were numerous options available to me. Beyond family and friends, I found that most retailers and service people were glad to help, often bending their standard way of doing things.

"This is my situation," I would say. "How would you solve it?" And, so it usually began, the collection of innovative ideas. We had groceries delivered and found services on the Internet that made house calls. Rich joked that a cottage industry was springing up around me. I had stopped seeing myself as a victim of cancer but rather as a survivor of life.

I began to use the clinic where I received infusions as my virtual office, anxious to keep a finger on the pulse of the business. My company was rumored to be in merger discussions with another telecommunications giant, meaning that all aspects of the business would be reassessed in light of an impending integration. I'd been through it before and knew that there would be excitement and new strategies, a blending of cultures and talent and functions. All leadership positions would be refocused on creating the new business and I wanted to be part of the metamorphosis.

Several work friends called to update me but I had no contact with my direct management and was feeling disenfranchised. There seemed to be a lot of scrambling as people positioned themselves for the new deal. I worried about the directors who had reported to me and who might not have a champion at the bargaining table. I worried about myself, outside of the loop, without input about potential options in the new environment. It was a bad time to be away from the business.

Unsure of exactly what I wanted, I was torn by the commitment to rebalance my priorities with a new protectiveness of my health. Then I remembered that when I was unsure if I would live, I realized that I had sacrificed precious time with the people I love in order to achieve a successful business career. It had paid off in terms of advancement and compensation. Now, contention between time with my family and my attention to the corporate world were being reexamined. I realized that my involvement in the business would have to be passive until I achieved my primary mission.

As we continued working the plan, Joanne, ever vigilant in her continuing research, had led to the discovery of new information that made her uncomfortable. While reading about the drugs being administered to me, she came across a possible effect of bleomycin that she thought I should discuss with Dr. Tseng.

"The information they gave you didn't mention anything about this, but look here. I looked it up in a medical library and found out it may cause a residual side effect that is serious and irreversible. The condition called pulmonary fibrosis is the growth of fibers in the lungs, a condition that would severely affect your ability to breathe. It's the kind of affliction that starts quietly but gets worse over time. It could radically change the quality of your life."

I imagined my lungs being clogged by the restricted passageways like roots of a tree that might choke a sewer line. The next day I conferred with Dr. Tseng.

"Yes, there have been some incidents of lung capacity impairment, but we administer only a very small amount. I don't think you have anything to worry about. But, if you'd feel better, we'll order a series of tests to be run so we know what's happening."

I appreciated Dr. Tseng's acknowledgment that this was not insignificant to me.

"I want to know. If it's going to happen, I want to know. And, if there's anything that can be done about it, I want to know about that too." I was seeking to make more informed decisions by getting all of the available data on critical subjects. I wanted to see options, even long shots, on each major decision. Even though the issues were frightening, I wanted to know.

I asked for lung tests to evaluate my pulmonary efficiency at passing oxygen to the blood, called oxygenation, which revealed some impairment in my lungs' performance. Dr. Tseng thought the condition was minimal and probably temporary. I wanted him to be right, but Joanne suggested that we hedge our bets.

"Now you need aerobic activity every day. No exceptions," she said.

She was asking a lot since I got winded just going up and down the stairs. Normally my little walks didn't range far from the house since my stomach was very unpredictable. But, Joanne's strategy sounded logical.

"If we do everything possible to expand the lung capacity through aerobic exercise, it may lessen the damage from the drug. I don't particularly care what you do but just keep moving. The thing you're most inclined to do—go to bed—is the worst thing you can do. We're talking about saving your lungs."

We developed daily charts of walking or stair-stepping starting with five minutes. Each week we tried to progress to the next five, for ten minutes, then fifteen minutes, then twenty, twenty-five. Sometimes, on very good days, it was as much as thirty. There were rare exceptions when the ravages of the chemotherapy prevented me from being out of bed. Otherwise, some form of aerobic activity was done daily.

Joanne wanted information about my blood to check for anomalies in the blood chemistry that might be nutrition based. Dr. Van Sickle agreeably ordered the additional blood work. I went to the lab for a special blood draw.

"Some patients never finish their treatment program." The nurse was sad when she said it, sad for the harshness of the treatment. "So many just give up."

At first I could not imagine how they could stop. After all, this was our chance to live. Halfway through, however, the thought of ending therapy became a powerfully seductive temptation. Just stop.

What kept me going was the data. We had documented my progress, tracking it against benchmarks that allowed us to make fact-based decisions. To the barometers, we added heart rate monitoring during aerobic exercise. Joanne reviewed the statistics with us, adjusting the program when my body indicated that it needed a different level of activity or nutritional sustenance. By late spring I could walk a block without stopping to catch my breath. By the beginning of May, ten weeks into therapy, I was training to improve my cardiovascular endurance. Where I had been hunched over because of my surgical incision, I was now strengthening my abdominal muscles through exercise. Incredibly, by the beginning of summer I was lifting free weights. I had entered a stage of Rebuilding.

"I think I'm ready for Mother to come out." And I called to invite her.

My mother, now in her seventies, improved her life after Daddy died. She was a wonderful teacher, retiring in El Paso, Texas, after thirty-three years of encouraging Latino kids to achieve their potential. Twenty years ago she married a kind, spiritual man who, unfortunately, had smoked heavily until middle age. Now in his eighties, he was suffering from throat cancer but refusing chemotherapy. It made him too sick, he said. Rich tried to keep Mother informed about my progress (without the gore), attempting to minimize her stress. She and I spoke on the phone every few days but we had stalled her attempts to come out for a visit. I was afraid that seeing me in my weakened condition would upset her. Mothers can see the truth.

Day-to-day living soon became a series of letting go of small burdens. I had noticed that, at times, I made strangers uncomfortable because I had no hair. I was very self-conscious about my looks and had gotten a nice wig. It functioned well when I felt I needed to look normal. However, besides itching my bald, sensitive head, it just wasn't me. I usually preferred to wear scarves or hats instead. One warm summer evening, Rich and I were dressing to go out with friends. I struggled and struggled with my wig, trying to get the right look and feel, thinking it appeared rather like it wasn't attached to my scalp at all, as though it were flying overhead and suddenly landed in this unlikely place.

"Wait. I just can't get this thing on right." I was frustrated.

Rich came over to me, pulled the wig off, and kissed my bald head.

"Ditch the wig. I love your head."

I never wore the wig again. I think back on it now with sadness that I felt so self-conscious about losing my hair during chemotherapy. It did make other people uncomfortable when I encountered them in public, but I just stopped caring about that. In actuality, we should be as proud as warriors wearing medals of courage, but the unfortunate truth is that our society finds it discomfiting.

While my immune system was disabled, I had become fastidious about controlling my exposure to germs. We replaced hand towels with paper towels and tried to sanitize surfaces where germs were most likely to incubate. If the children were at all contagious they could not visit me. By the middle of summer, my white blood count normalized, indicating that my immune function was being restored. This improved condition meant that Katie, our three-year-old granddaughter just recovering from a cold, could finally come over with her mom, Kelly.

"Gramma—what happened to your hair?" Katie was seeing me bald for the first time. Her eyes huge, she froze in her tracks, unsure whether or not to approach.

"I took some medicine that made it fall out." I tried to sound light, disguising my concern that she would be afraid.

"Katie, look, it's coming back. See the little fuzz? Come feel it." I bent down and took her hand, and together we rubbed the soft down that had begun to present itself.

"Why did you do it, Gramma Net?"

"Because sometimes we need medicine to get well even if it isn't very pleasant. Just like when you take cough medicine that doesn't taste good. So, now I'm getting better and I get new hair that feels just like the fur on a baby chick. What do you think of that?"

"I'm glad you're better, Gramma Net. And I like your new hair."

It was during this time that Kelly borrowed some expensive antique earrings for a special occasion. When she returned them in the case, I had not looked at them immediately. It was not until weeks later that I noticed one was missing. I was reluctant to tell her but felt that the missing earring might have fallen into the suitcase or her clothes and could be found. Although I tried not to upset her, she immediately began tearing her house apart, panicked at the thought of losing something irreplaceable. Finally, her husband found the stray jewelry in the car, the victim of little Katie's curiosity. Distraught, Kelly rushed the earring to me and was clearly shaken by the time I saw her.

"It's just a thing," I told her in a vain attempt to calm her down. "It is no different from any rock in the street. Somebody just said it had value and everybody believed it. Trust me—it's not worth this much emotion. You should only get this upset over the family or your health or something really important. Honestly, all the time I was in the hospital I never once thought about my jewelry."

She did not seem consoled. She could not see what was clear to me: when you stand to lose it all, your choices become very simple.

14

Dimensions Of Healing

In the beginning, I thought I'd feel better as soon as I stopped getting infusions, but after we were well into the process, we discovered that I was quite mistaken. My chemotherapy seemed to have a cumulative effect, and, for me, the worst two weeks were those following the last infusions. Shortly after, however, I did get better. Slowly, but steadily, I began to reclaim my life and my health, bit by bit.

It was the middle of July, when summer finally came to Oregon, that my amazing recovery began. My nausea let up in stages, as did many other side effects, all of which diminished day by day. At a fairly rapid rate, symptoms that I feared I might have for the rest of my life began to disappear. I worried that my reflux would never be normal again and then it was. One day, I noticed that it just went away. Just like that.

I began sleeping through the night more and more often. This significantly reduced my fatigue, as well as Rich's. Other small signs of recovery began popping up around our lives, such as the absence of a pharmacy sitting on my nightstand as my medications dropped off. I could feel the healing going on inside and I sensed a cleansing of my veins and arteries. I dreamed of toxins being purged from every pore of my body, their job completed, like doughboys climbing out of foxholes on the Western Front, battered and bruised, but finally going home. Well done!

As soon as the medications dissolved or discharged, my senses of taste and smell normalized. I could cook or go out to dinner without being assaulted by an aroma that became twisted by the therapy. My appetite returned. I knew I was better the day "chocolate" sounded like a great idea. I reclaimed my kitchen and, armed with my new knowledge, I tried to make choices for a healthier lifestyle.

No longer easily winded, I began walking with our two dogs, strong, high-energy bird hunters who prefer an elevated pace. My aerobic capacity improved and my energy level increased. The pains in my stomach went away and my joints no longer ached. Rich and I started going to movies in the evening again and to concerts and plays. More laughter could be heard around the house. By the middle of August, I returned to my job and traveled to a business meeting at corporate headquarters—without my wig.

Recovery, however, involved more than the physical changes I went through as my body began to shake off the ravages of treatment. It involved my psychological wellness as well. One day during the summer I mentioned to Dennis that I could only use alcohol-free lotions because the chemotherapy created skin sensitivity.

"When exactly will you stop thinking of yourself as a chemotherapy patient and begin living in recovery? Do you realize that you stopped treatment weeks ago?"

His words fell on me with a thud. I was still living in a reality that no longer existed for me, yet I had no sense of moving on. Although we had rejoiced at not having to go back for infusions and I was feeling better, I had not changed my thinking about the thousands of daily decisions that had been part of the last five months. It was finally over.

"It's like getting out of prison. I guess I knew I didn't have to wear the uniform anymore but I hadn't let go of all the little things we were so obsessive about for so long." As I spoke the words, the reality of being free began to sink in. Now I could shed the shroud of sickness that I had lived with and even gotten comfortable with. I wasn't that sick person anymore.

My hair grew back in the fall. Strangely, it wasn't that important to me anymore. I still find it curious that I had cried so deeply when I lost it, perhaps because it symbolized this inexplicable disaster that had befallen me. I had avoided looking in the mirror during the long months of chemotherapy because the person reflected there was not the person in my mind. What I have learned since is that the person looking back can be better than the image. If a person is true and just, looks for the beauty in the world, and shares love with others, then that person is beautiful.

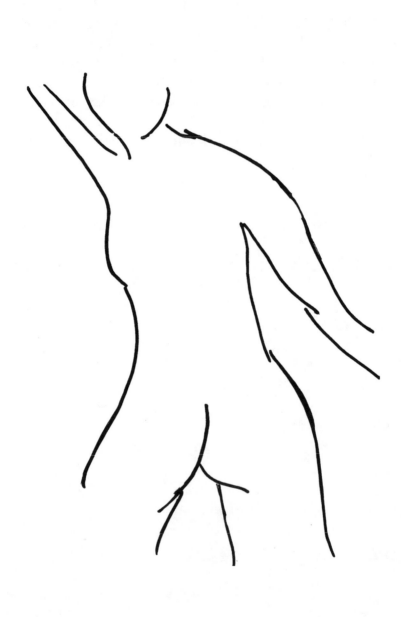

15

The Lessons

There were times when I was in chemotherapy that I thought dying would be better, but it's not. Some people choose not to endure chemotherapy because they fear the harshness of the treatments. Some begin and never finish. I believe that we managed the negative side effects of my treatments by utilizing the natural resources of the body and the mind to support and enhance the medical program. This approach produced a synergy from three powerful forces working together to achieve a successful recovery. First was the established medical model of treatment. Not only did this form the foundation of the structure; it was the crux of survival. Next was the psychosocial and spiritual element that gave me the hope and the resolve to live. And, finally, the physical component, comprised of fitness and nutrition, provided the reserves to propel me toward wellness. Individually, each of these elements was a critical factor of survival; together they created a whole that was greater than the sum of its parts. I believe it worked. First, I got better, and then I got well—very, very well.

I know that the holistic approach we took had a profound effect on my outcome. It helped me fight the disease, both physically and psychologically. I contracted no contagious illnesses, such as colds or flu, even though my immune system was crippled. Anti-cancer drugs can inflict lasting damage on the skin, yet my skin was smooth and supple again a year after recovery. Not only was my body able to sustain itself during this long battle; it built a reservoir to restore the systems of the body, thus allowing them to function at optimal levels under the circumstances.

Chemotherapy is an opportunity to survive cancer. Although our story describes the difficulty of my journey, it is meant to pass along our discoveries that made it less so. It was the right decision for us. Rich and I believe that choosing alternative therapy in lieu of proven medical treatments is very foolish and dangerous. We investigated alternative treatments that might assist advanced stage cancers or cancers for which there was no effective treatment. The credible studies were those based on peer review by the medical community and published in respected medical journals. Some of these therapies, known as "adjuvant" (helpful) therapies are being tested as ways to augment and enhance medical treatments. Some studies involve alternative or naturopathic treatments.

Assuming full accountability for my situation was the most critical decision that I made in the process. I viewed the physicians as technicians responsible for the functioning medical part of the solution, not the total solution. They are wonderful doctors and nurses, sympathetic and competent, but they represented only one aspect of what was happening to me. I chose to control many variables that impacted my quality of life: diet, exercise, and psychological and spiritual strength, which directly affected my ability to cope with the illness. I observed some patients at the cancer clinic who passively endured the therapy, relinquishing responsibility for their treatment to the health care professionals. Looking back now, I have no evidence that our results were better, or that those patients were mistaken in their approach. I only know that it would never have been enough for me. It was illogical to me not to do everything possible to improve my situation, to be responsive versus reactive to my predicament. I believe that my body was stronger for it, and I know that my spirit was.

The detailed, coarse description of my experience is not intended to discourage others from therapy. My experience was difficult because of my unique treatment plan and my post-surgical situation. However, some patients who were on different combinations of drugs experienced fewer side effects, some virtually none at all. In addition, new anti-nausea medications are demonstrating great success for most chemotherapy patients. Given the same choices again, I would choose to do it.

Psychological health was essential. I have not met one person with cancer who hasn't experienced rage, fear, grief, depression, and confusion. Psychotherapy helped me to feel the honesty of my emotions without being overwhelmed by them. I had a right to feel angry, depressed, confused, and very scared, but I also had choices. Therapy helped me to stay focused on things that improved my recovery. It was also important for our friends and family to be able to deal with the emotional trauma of having a loved one ill with cancer. The caregiver is too often forgotten, overshadowed by the patient.

Communication was vital at every step in the process. In the beginning, there was so much information that I couldn't remember all the details. Much of the language was technical medical jargon and I wasn't always sure I understood exactly what was being said. Particularly in the beginning, it felt like we were living in informational quicksand. The journal we kept for doctors' phone numbers became expanded to include follow-up issues and questions and it helped to keep information straight. When doctors gave us bad or difficult news, I was not always able to process it, so writing it down helped me to understand later what had been said. Also, complicated procedures were sometimes confusing and I might ask the doctor to write down the details in the journal for reference at another time. Health care professionals devoted to treating cancer talk to patients every day who are facing life-threatening situations for the first time in their lives; they expect to be questioned.

We trusted and respected our medical team and we felt confident that they were solidly in our corner fighting the battle with us. They further confirmed that our confidence was well placed when they responded to our inquiries by helping us to understand the chemistry of healing and supported our efforts to contribute to a positive conclusion.

Spirituality came to us early in our journey, strengthened by the undying faith of my sister Sylvia. I prayed more during this time than I ever had before in my life and received comfort as well as strength. I also believe we had miracles bestowed upon us. Perhaps in guiding the surgeon's hand during a complicated surgical procedure, perhaps inspiring the reclassification of the cancer to that of a treatable type, we believe that miracles did happen.

Some months after surgery I had a follow-up visit with my surgeon, Dr. Swartz. He told me of another case where he was called in for consultation, another woman diagnosed with pancreatic cancer.

"I was confused because her tumor was not in the right position for pancreatic. Then I remembered your case and pursued her history, only to find that she had also been treated for ovarian cancer some years ago. I guess there's some similarity in the cell structure and that's why they thought it was pancreatic but it wasn't. It was just like yours, granulosa cell. Had it not been for your case, I don't think we'd have caught it."

For her, there was a miracle.

Rich and I had many moments of the awareness of God. Most are very personal. The most powerful was at the end of my therapy when we met with Dr. Tseng for a very frank discussion about my future. We wanted to make practical decisions about our projected time together. He surprised us with news that any recurrence of the cancer should grow at the same rate as the last, ten to twelve years. That was when we learned that we would likely have more than five years together. I had been so fixated on my five-year goal that this news completely changed our time horizon by doubling it. I believe that getting my life back was a gift from God. But I also believe that like all gifts, it was in our hands to steward.

There were times when we saw others with heavier burdens and we were humbled. We were blessed in so many ways, and we counted our blessings often during the journey. We were surrounded and supported by love, that which we had for each other and the love of our family and friends. Of the many things I experienced with cancer, I never suffered from loneliness.

Most importantly, we have faith and we are blindly, single-mindedly, optimistic about our future.

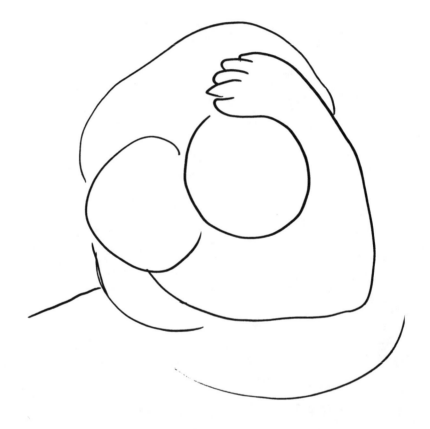

16

Choices

Throughout the summer Mother had tried to schedule a visit. She had been anxious to see me for months but afraid to leave her husband who was weak from not eating due to his own throat cancer. All the while, he insisted on making the trip from El Paso with her, refusing to be left behind. Finally, we picked a time in the early fall when the weather in Oregon is spectacular, hoping he would be well enough to travel by then. However, as the day approached, he was hospitalized with pneumonia and within a week the fine old gentleman passed away.

He was a sweet and simple man with a generous heart. Until the time he became ill, he sang and played his guitar to entertain elderly invalids at a neighborhood nursing home. He had loved my mother and all of us, but it was the children who owned his heart. As a young man he had adopted two orphans, a niece and nephew, and raised them alongside his own kids. A surrogate father to anyone who needed one, he counseled neighborhood boys about the dangers of gangs and the merits of school. His last years had been spent as a loving grandfather, happily teaching Sylvia's children the wisdom of his considerable life through games and songs and parables. I had thought it curious that he always kept a bicycle pump on his front porch, since he had no bike. It had been there for the neighborhood kids.

It was when we went to Texas for the funeral that I saw Mother for the first time since my illness. She was so nervous, fearful that I might be dying too. She had been torn between caring for her husband and coming to Portland to care for me, but she had made the right choice. Immediately relieved that I looked strong and healthy, she allowed her fears to be put away. Now, she could concentrate on burying her husband.

I was surprised to see several teenage boys from the neighborhood among the many people who came to the service. As they said their tearful goodbyes, it was clear that they would miss the kind old fellow who had cared about them and had been their friend. I was moved by their open affection and I wondered, in that moment, what children would cry that way for me. I then made a choice.

My last several years as a corporate executive had demanded that I be away nearly seventy percent of the time. During our darkest moments, it was the only thing that Rich and I regretted about our life together—that I had been gone so much. That absence was no longer acceptable. So, even though accommodations were made for me to return to the business, I accepted an early retirement to do the things that I love: enjoy my family, work on things that intrigue me, leave a better world for our children, and write my book.

My original intent was to write a guidebook for families like us, surprised by the impact of cancer, the kind of book we wished had been on the shelf when we went looking. I had in mind a kind of "how to" from a patient's point of view, with lists and clues, pointers for those stunned by a diagnosis of catastrophic illness.

Then, within just a few months, two events occurred that changed my story . . . and forever changed my life.

17

New Lessons From An Old Teacher

Walter and Gloria had remained friends with me since the mid-seventies when we had met in Washington, D.C. We now saw each other every couple of years and it was always wonderful and full and too short for the long distance between us.

In 1996 Walter was diagnosed with pancreatic cancer. Gloria got him into Johns Hopkins University Hospital where he underwent radical surgery to remove a deadly tumor. It seemed that he had recovered so well, bouncing back strong and vigorous, as we always expected him to be. He took an early retirement, threw his vigor into revitalizing Old Town Manassas and his antiques business, and enjoying life with Gloria. He was happier than he had ever been in his life. As soon as I could travel, Rich and I had gone to Washington to visit Walter and Gloria and celebrate our miraculous recoveries.

A few months later, while working on a first draft of this book, I received a call from my old friend who had one more lesson for me.

"Hi, Annette. It's Walter." The Boston accent was his but the voice was older, somber, different from the teasing voice I had heard less than a year ago. A born extrovert, he always sounded so effervescent on the phone. I used to tease him about it.

"Always a smile, Walter Delisle," I used to rhyme when he answered my calls.

But today was different.

"Walter?"

The phone felt cold in my hands and goose bumps went up my arms.

"Walter . . . what's up?" I began to feel nervous for some reason—the sound in his voice, perhaps.

"Well, I was having some problems and they couldn't find it at first, so they sent me back to Johns Hopkins."

The pause told me more than the words that followed.

"My cancer . . . it's back again. They did an exploratory and it looks like it's all over the place. This time they say I have about six months to live. So, I'm calling to let you know."

"Wait. Walter, wait a minute." I was hardly able to process, my thinking stuck on the finality of his words. I sat down on the bed, the phone trembling in my hands. This wasn't the way it was supposed to happen.

"Isn't there some kind of treatment? What about alternative medicine?"

My mind scrambled for a shred of information that might be useful.

"There's new information about homeopathic therapies, studies on the effects of alternative therapies that might help. Or . . . or clinical trials. Have you looked into clinical trials, Walter?"

I felt swept into a rushing river, grasping at any passing branch that might keep me from being washed away.

"We have to do something, right? There must be something," my voice desperate now, pleading with my old friend with the big personality and the bigger heart not to give up just like that, without a fight. Not Walter.

"We've been at Johns Hopkins, Annette. The simple fact is that there is no treatment for this cancer. None. Heck, I should have died the first time. It's a miracle that I'm here now. Supposedly, I'm one of the longest living survivors of this particular kind of cancer as it is. Besides, going through chemo, if it had any impact at all, it would only extend my life a little, give me a little more time, but it would make me sick for most of it. I decided that if they can't cure it, then I want to spend the rest of my days living the best way that I can for whatever time I have left."

I was astounded by his acceptance of the fatal prognosis. He did not sound angry but perhaps sad, and yet in a peaceful way.

"I can't believe it. You looked great the last time I saw you."

Rich and I had compared notes with Walter and Gloria, amazed by the parallels between our incredible journeys of cancer recovery. We laughed and cried, amazed that Walter and I had each dodged such a deadly bullet. He was so full of life then, a strong, energetic man just fifty-seven years old, with bright blue eyes and bushy salt-and-pepper hair. And a huge smile. Always a huge smile. One of those smiles that opens wide like a book to reveal its secrets inside.

"When did all this happen?"

"I'd been having problems for four or five months with fatigue and stomach pains when I ate. My gastrointestinal specialist identified an iron deficiency and thought it was a secondary reaction to my surgery. After two iron infusions, I felt more energetic but the stomach pains kept recurring. They did everything: gastroscopy, colonoscopy, and fluoroscopy, as well as my yearly CT scan, but nothing indicated a recurrence. They thought it was from adhesions—you know how scar tissue sometimes gums things up in there."

"Yes, I know."

"But, unfortunately it's the cancer, back again. We just found out that there's a new kind of scan that might have told us sooner, but for me it was too late to even consider options. Then again, I'm not sure it would have made any difference. The fact is: I'm gonna die."

I did not want to process what I was hearing, that every stone had been overturned. But I knew Walter, knew that he had done a thorough job of examining the situation and he had made his decision.

"They just don't know very much about pancreatic cancer. Statistically, the risk increases when you're older or a smoker, but I'm not that old and I never smoked. In fact, I've been in very good health all my life until now. I guess it's just my time."

"Isn't there anything, anything at all?"

"Heck, the five-year survival rate for *treatable* pancreatic cancer is only five percent, Annette. We put up a good fight but it looks like cancer's gonna win this round."

I closed my eyes and tried to picture his face, as serene as his voice was calm. Finally accepting, I asked him how he was dealing with this new turn of events.

"You know, I feel pretty lucky. Most people never know when they're going to die. I get to make all my plans, get my affairs in order. Gloria and I can make decisions about her future. We just got back from Mexico from our favorite vacation spot. I get to say goodbye to all my friends and family, make sure nothing is left unsaid. How great is that?"

Silently I wept, unable to speak.

"I think I'm fortunate to have the chance to make my own arrangements for the things I care about. I've even planned the funeral, including the program. Gloria and I worked on it together. It's the least I can do for her. She'd been taking such great care of me; that's why I made it this far."

"Walter, my heart is breaking. I'm so sorry. I don't know what to say except I love you."

"That's all you need to say. Look, I'm at peace with it. I believe God has a master plan and I have a role in it somewhere. It's just not my privilege to know what it is. Who am I to second-guess Him? You know, I should have died the first time, nearly five years ago. So, I don't ask myself, 'Why am I gonna die?' I ask, 'Why did I live?' There must be a reason. When I get up every morning, I get dressed and go out and basically approach every day as though it's the most important day of my life. I try to stay open to the possibilities, you know, just in case today's the day that something will happen that will really make a difference in the world."

"What can I do for you?"

"Don't worry about me; I'm going to be fine. Just check in on Gloria from time to time. The worst part of all this is my leaving the woman who loved me more than I deserved. I just hate leaving her." Gloria had been married to Walter for thirty-seven years. Soon she would be a widow.

I sank into a terrible sadness that went deep, deep inside of me. I wanted to hold him, feel the life in him, and to not believe that it was true. Walter would die in just a few months. Yet, when I went back to see him a few weeks later, it was he who comforted me. To the end, he had the biggest shoulders in town.

A short time later, Walter held his own Irish wake in New England where he grew up. He shared his philosophy of life, coaching anyone who would listen to his ideas about changing the world for the better. Lifelong friends and long lost relatives all came to toast and roast their old friend. He said it was one hell of a party—but he was not done.

"Annette, you know as well as anyone, I've always had an opinion about how people should do things. Now, I guess I have to step up. I don't see that I have a choice. The way I see it, I get to show people how to die with cancer, how to do the right things with the time you have left. I wish I could show other people how to capture the really important moments, you know, like making a kid laugh or kissing someone you care about. How to love right to the end. I think that's why I lived, to show people first to be square with God and next to be square with your own heart—every day."

Walter spent the next few months by filling the days with as much as anyone could possibly handle.

"I wish I had lived every day as if it were my last day. Who knows? I might have been president!" and he would laugh easily and honestly, making anyone around him laugh with him.

Two months later in February, when I went back for another visit, Gloria and I had to track him down on his cell phone. He was a very busy man. Every day Walter jumped on a full schedule of commitments. He remained active in local politics, attending every town meeting his health would allow. He spent his days fixated on arranging their affairs to accommodate Gloria when she would be handling everything alone. Business and personal matters were streamlined, partnerships unraveled. He redesigned the antiques business to suit Gloria's needs, a final tribute to the woman he had loved all his adult life and now would leave behind. I asked Gloria what the doctors had to say about his condition. Shouldn't he slow down?

"First of all, he won't do it. It doesn't matter what the doctors say, he's up every day really early. He dresses, goes out to breakfast downtown to catch up on town politics, and then to his shop to take care of business. If I'm lucky, he'll come home for a short nap after lunch. But, sometimes he doesn't; sometimes he just keeps going.

"I took a leave from the hospital to be home with him, but half the time I can't find him. He's in meetings and doing deals. He's just pushing himself to get everything done before . . ."

"Aren't you worried, afraid he'll collapse? What if he has a problem?"

"The doctor says he can do whatever he's able to do. I was worried that he was sapping the last of his energy and that he would fail faster. But, the doctors say it's possible that it might have the opposite effect: his drive may keep him alive longer. Anyway, there's no slowing him down. You try." The tone in her voice laid bare her emotional and physical exhaustion, yet in many ways her pride in the man she had chosen as a life partner.

The next morning Walter was off to see to his chores and couldn't wait for us to rally. We caught up with him at lunch. Half a dozen townspeople were milling around his table at the local restaurant. He was holding court.

"They made him the Unofficial Mayor of Old Town Manassas," Gloria informed me as we both stood watching, baffled by his rigorous pace, and I knew this was his finest hour. "In recognition of all those years when he kept pushing for his dream of a picturesque, historic business community with restaurants, galleries, and, of course, antiques. He was the real force behind the revitalization of Old Town. It wouldn't be what it is today were it not for him. So, last week he was officially appointed unofficial mayor. All the people from the town came and gave public comments to the Mayor and City Council on his appointment. Some were hilarious, but they all ended thanking Walt for all the things he's done."

He was so very proud. Now there was no doubt that he had improved his part of the world. Many years from now some stranger who knew nothing of the man would cherish the work he had left behind.

By April, he had started counting "Plus Months."

"They said I'd be gone by March, so every month from now on is a Plus Month. April is Plus One."

Rich took me back to see him then for what we knew would be the last time. He was much thinner and very tired but still stubborn as hell. He had just received further evidence of his value to the city. The Walter J. Delisle Park, a beautiful playground for children, was built on a shady corner lot near his home and dedicated in his honor. Walter proudly walked me around the park, showing me each unique part, explaining why it was special to him. In typical Walter style, he had inserted himself in the planning, design, and execution, even helping to prepare the site. He contributed so much effort to the project that friends began to joke that he didn't really have cancer and they suspected a hidden ploy.

"I told Gloria that if I don't go soon the city's going to take my park away. So, I'm thinking about sleeping out here so, in case they try, they'll have to carry me out first." And he lay down on the slide, crossing his arms over his chest as though lying in state, laughing while his grandsons jumped all over him.

For the next two months, he carefully tended the gardens in his park, reveling in the legacy he would leave behind. On any day he could be seen flagging down friends to come pull the stubborn weeds from the blossoming borders or leaning against the lamp-posts arguing the merits of zoning changes in his beloved Virginia community. He showed his grandchildren where they could come to talk to him whenever they needed him, promising them that he would still be there even after he was gone. Vowing never to spend a day in bed, he lived beyond the expectations of his doctors, shocking the hospice nurse because he was gardening the day she came for her first home visit.

As he lived his life, so he ended it. True to his promise, he got up each day and crammed every moment with the things he believed were important, as one might pack a trunk for a very long voyage, stowing in each corner another cherished memory. That is until the Fourth of July, 2001, the day he died. How fitting that he passed on as fireworks lit the sky, as though showing him the way up to heaven.

Walter was right; so many people never figure it out until it's too late. What he taught me in the end was that I am lucky as well as he, to know how precious my time is here. Walter helped me to understand that what we do during our brief stay here must have meaning, or it will be as though we never happened at all. We each have a lifetime of opportunities to create beauty, to make someone happy, to find truth. We just never know when that lifetime is up.

I also believe that love plays such an important role in our lives. Walter felt blessed because he had achieved a life of incredible love, the love he shared with his family and friends and the lifetime of love between himself and Gloria. It is the same love that comforts Gloria now that she is alone.

Goodbye, my old teacher . . . I will miss you, my dear old friend.

18

A Further Test Of Faith

It was December 2000 and we began preparing for another big family Christmas. We would count our blessings, love each other, and be thankful for my restored health. Then, within days, it happened. We received another shock, the cruelest of them all.

The phone rang late that night as with most calls of bad news. It was Cindy, my stepdaughter from my former marriage. Cindy was fourteen years old when I became her stepmother at age twenty-eight. She and I stumbled our way through her rebellious teenage years, bonding in the process. We had reconnected over the years and had become particularly close since my illness. Rich and I had visited Cindy and her husband Rob in California the previous spring and that summer they and their three children visited us in Oregon.

"It's Justin." Her fear clung to the sound of her son's name, bringing me instantly awake. "A brain tumor."

No, no, no.

"He was fine, perfectly fine. Then, the other night he stumbled when he got up from dinner. We laughed and I thought he just had puppy feet. But, the next morning when he couldn't keep his balance, I told Rob I had this feeling something was seriously wrong." Her voice was trembling and I knew she was shaking.

"I'm so scared," her words resonating with my forgotten feelings. I knew that fear, the one that goes so deep that it permeates the very marrow of your bones.

Once the hospital in San Jose had discovered the tumor on Justin's brain stem, he was rushed to the University of California at San Francisco Hospital where specialists in pediatric brain tumors were evaluating him. I was to meet the family there.

On the flight to California I thought a lot about Cindy, remembering how she had changed when Justin was born. He became her reason for living from the time he was in her womb. Still in disbelief myself, I tried to imagine what terror she must be feeling. She had felt it before.

It was 1989, when the baby was about six months old, that the last big earthquake crippled the Bay Area. It cost several lives and billions of dollars in damage, destroying homes and business from Oakland to Santa Cruz, San Francisco to San Jose. The earthquake was a disaster of Biblical proportions. It was then that she almost lost him.

Cindy worked in Palo Alto while Baby Justin stayed home in the daily care of relatives in the Santa Cruz Mountains. When the quake hit, it dismantled all public infrastructures: bridges collapsed, phone lines were down, power was out, and emergency services were overwhelmed. The wreckage was everywhere. Citizens who were safe were ordered to stay put. Chaos had set in.

To get to Justin, Cindy would have to cross the San Francisco Peninsula and fight her way up the mountain. She assessed what it would take to find him then, through pure determination, acquired boots, flashlight, batteries, rope, and water. She started out by car, making her way toward home—the epicenter of the disaster. Highways were impassable; traffic was gnarled and being turned back from the direction she was headed. Still she kept going. When she could no longer drive, she walked. When she found someone who was sympathetic, she hitched a ride. More than once officials tried to turn her around.

"You'll have to arrest me." She was going to find her son.

As she got halfway up the mountain, she found the road completely gone with no place to even walk. She reverted to hiking through the forest. Homes throughout the area were destroyed, their foundations broken like matchsticks, the structures crushed without the underlying support. Some fell off footings and were still slipping into gaping crevices in the earth as she passed them. Finally, after hours of breaking barrier after barrier, she came upon ruins of the structure where Justin was being cared for and it was then that she panicked. But, miraculously, the family had narrowly escaped the collapse and was sheltered nearby with the baby. Justin was safe.

Cindy had become a terrific mother. Finally finding her true north, she embraced the role with immeasurable devotion. She is great at it, the kind of mom that is always aware of her children. They were her reason for being, Justin and his sisters, six-year-old Kelly and Allison, almost one.

The doctors in San Francisco proceeded to tell us the worst. The biopsy confirmed that it was a brain stem glioma, a hideous disease that affects only children. This rare cancer afflicts only 330 children in this country each year. Justin was one of them. The alien growth intertwined its deadly fibers through the brain stem of a healthy, happy kid, short-circuiting his motor and sensory functions. It was growing fast, the onslaught of symptoms appearing literally overnight.

We were then told, in sympathetic but direct terms, that the tumor was inoperable and the cancer was fatal. There was no way to save him.

"We can give him radiation treatment and try to contain the tumor, but it's very aggressive and it will eventually shut his body down. We lose most children with this cancer within the year."

We asked if there was anything else we could do—clinical trials or experimental studies. We didn't care how slim the possibilities. We believed in doing the impossible. We would do it, whatever it was. Even if the odds were one tenth of one percent, we needed to hold onto our hope. Before this, Justin was healthy and strong, we reasoned. Why couldn't he be the one that beat the odds? Some child will be the breakthrough child. Why not him?

There was a slim possibility that he could be helped with experimental treatment at Stanford University Hospital. A clinical trial was being conducted to test the effectiveness of using chemotherapy to make the tumor less resistant to the radiation. Normally the level of radiation administered is limited in intensity to prevent brain damage. The combined effect of the therapies should cause the tumor to burn from the middle outward, thus causing it to retract its grip on the brain cells and, hopefully, restore their connections. It had shown promise in a few cases, extending a child's life and improving his quality of life in the process . . . for a while.

Long enough for a miracle?

In a matter of hours, Justin had experienced frightening things happening to his body, as though some evil villain were throwing switches that controlled his sight, his hearing, and his ability to swallow and to breathe. Everything was strange to him; nothing was the way it should be. Cindy had told him it was cancer that was making him sick and now he was waiting for someone to help him. That's what hospitals are for, isn't it? To make people well who were sick? To save people from dying? Instead of making him better, the doctors were having hushed discussions with the family away from his room where he couldn't hear. That made him more and more nervous.

"He wants you to tell him how to beat cancer." Cindy had told Justin of my recovery the previous year. He knew cancer was deadly and he thought I was pretty amazing to win such a terrifying battle. Surely there was something I knew that soon he would know. Then he would be better too.

"Can you talk to him so he won't be afraid?" She could not mask her dread from him. She needed me to find a truth that she could live with and that he would accept.

I sat on the bed and took his hand. As I looked at it, I saw the hand of a little boy, soft and smooth, without the calluses and scars of life's experience. There was nothing to temper the pain or fear or confusion. These hands were innocent and untouched. They knew no tools, had no frame of reference. I wondered how he could possibly comprehend what would be happening to him.

"The doctors have a plan to help you, Justin. They're going to use radiation to zap the tumor. It's very precise technology, just like a laser. It's amazing how they can pinpoint exactly where to hit it. The idea is to blast the tumor right in the middle, knocking it out so it will stop messing with your brain." He looked at Cindy, knowing she could not lie to him. Sensing her agony, he began to cry. I held him and continued explaining what we had agreed he could know.

"Justin, the best experts in the world are right there at Stanford. They want you there because they're the ones doing the research into this exact cancer. That's all they do there—work with kids just like you. But, they need your help, Justin. You'll be doing some uncomfortable things, but they need you to hang in there. The most important thing for you to do is to keep fighting. You have to remember, don't give up the fight. Your job will be to think about getting better every day."

"If I get better will I be in your book? Then we could tell everyone how to beat cancer, couldn't we?"

Yes, my angel, we'll tell them. We'll tell them all.

None of the lessons of my experience seemed important now. I was ashamed, ashamed of being proud of my ability to conquer my illness. All the while, like some monster in a movie that refuses to die, the antagonist in this story had lain in wait, nested in the body of a cherub. On the flight home. I felt adrift in a sea of sadness. I was lost in despair. How could I believe that my God could allow this to happen to a beautiful boy who would never become a man? I prayed for understanding and begged for a miracle.

Just one more.

At once I felt guilty for having lived, knowing that he would die. Was there no way to trade? Can you not make a deal with God as Faust made a deal with the devil? Couldn't we exchange one life for another?

As Justin entered the clinical trial at Stanford, Cindy and Rob restructured their lives to meet the overwhelming demands of daily medical procedures, Justin's rapidly failing health, and the parenting of Justin's two younger sisters. We were told that after six weeks of radiation, Justin should expect a "honeymoon" period, a time of near normal function. In all cases, however, the cancer had reawakened after a time and continued its deadly mission.

"His doctor said the radiation almost always shrinks the tumor. The treatments will really wipe him out but we want him to have some normal use of his body again." Cindy was hanging on to the shred of optimism.

"The way he is right now, he can't talk on the phone to his friends, he can't see very well, and he's losing his ability to walk. His best friend has been great and comes over all the time. But, otherwise, Justin's pretty isolated. We just want him to have some good days. You know, just to be a little boy again."

I did not know that there was a grief deeper than any I had felt in fifty years, but there was, and I was drowning in it. Emotionally devastated and despondent, I asked Dennis to help me bare the incredible anguish that had overtaken me. I couldn't work during the day and couldn't sleep without pills.

"When it's coming on, let it come. It is the deepest, most honest feeling one ever has. Give yourself time to feel it, as painful as it is. Then, you need to put it aside so you can feel other feelings. You need to balance the terrible pain you're feeling or you'll get sick. Your immune system is still pretty vulnerable. Rich is worried about you and I think he has a right to be. It's okay to think about Justin, just not all the time, at every meal, in every conversation. You need to talk about other things in your life. Believe me, you'll be more help to them if you're whole. Every week, you and Rich go out and do something that is fun. And, try to work out a reasonable schedule of visits to California at times when you'll be the most help. Use your tools, remember? If they need help, help them find it. You don't have to do it yourself."

He was right. There were resources through the hospital and various associations. Some were well organized; others were not. Also, support organizations offered any number of services, such as kinder care for siblings or tickets to sporting events. The challenge for Cindy and Rob was the coordination and management of the potential resources given Justin's medical needs and the growing list of agencies and departments associated with his treatments. There was no clearinghouse and many details that would have made the experience less complicated were overlooked. For example, when Justin needed a wheelchair, no one was told that his long waiting periods would be more comfortable if he had a recliner model. Not knowing that one existed, Cindy and Rob had gotten the wrong kind.

Justin endured the six weeks of dual treatments while his parents prayed for signs of improvement. They were distraught, begging for more time, yet devastated by what they could see happening to their son. The transformation was shocking.

"How's he doing?" I talked with Cindy every other day, between treatments and doctor appointments and shots.

"It's so hard because he's just a boy and these are devastating feelings for anyone, much less a child. He never complains when we're in treatment, which the nurses said is very unusual. I wanted to know if he was repressing his feelings, so I asked him if he was angry, and he said, 'Why? What good would that do, Mom?' He's doing a lot better than I am 'cause I'm angry, damn angry. I just don't know who to be angry at."

About every three weeks I went to California to help Cindy, alternating visits with her sister Teri. Rich was understandably worried about my ability to sustain the emotional stress and the physical demands. On my last visit, after a twelve-hour delay, I had been stranded at San Francisco Airport until the next morning. Rapidly overtaken by fatigue, I knew I was getting sick. Worse, I didn't know how to impact the outcome of this unbelievable nightmare. I felt helpless and useless.

Also, I knew that if this was devastating to me, then what about Cindy? Rob and Cindy? I prayed as much for them not to crumble under this terrible weight. Theirs was a greater madness.

As I prepared for my next trip south, I asked Dennis to help me to help Justin. I feared that I had nothing, nothing at all to give him. What could I possibly do to help?

"Justin is being asked to comprehend death and he hardly knows what life is. The more isolated he becomes, the more he'll ponder the idea of death and dying. The problem is children aren't emotionally experienced and they have a harder time coping with such intense feelings and thoughts. It might be too much for him and he could give up. And, if he gives up, well . . . he loses the battle.

"Remember how you felt refreshed after your friends' visits? Try to give him the same kind of emotional break. He needs to step away from it or it will overtake him. Have Cindy pick a time every day when he'll have a 'laugh hour,' with funny movies or anything that might make him laugh. Have his friends send funny cards or jokes. Tell them it's a contest and give prizes for the loudest laugh."

"And, for Cindy?"

"Don't give up or he'll give up. She should try to keep him thinking about winning, about getting better, and the only way she can do that is by not giving up hope herself. The mind can make the body do miraculous things. And, that's what we need now, a miracle.

"Every day I ask God to give me an intuitive thought as to how I might view a situation and what my response, if any, should be. Tell Cindy to keep praying and not to lose her faith. She needs the kind of strength that only comes from God."

She had asked me on the phone if she was foolish for not accepting the inevitable. No, I had told her, no, of course not. We couldn't give up hope. Not now.

"When will I know?"

"You'll know."

The tenacious tumor resisted the treatments; there was no honeymoon. Following radiation, Justin became worse. The crippling tumor now interfered with all of his senses: his ability to hear, see, taste, touch, and smell all malfunctioned simultaneously. He was confined to bed or a wheelchair. He was now completely dependant on others for virtually everything. He was losing ground and he knew it.

"Am I going to die?" he had asked one day when it was finally apparent to us all that there was no more hope.

Yes, Justin. But don't be afraid of death because it's only a door to a beautiful place. A place where everything is wonderful, with no pain or sadness. A place with God.

"A place without cancer?"

Yes, a place where you will be well.

After my last trip to see him, I was overtaken by intense anger, a fury brought on by the futility of prayers and procedures that had wasted the last few weeks of Justin's world.

"It's not your choice who lives and who dies."

Dennis knew everything else. Why didn't he know this? Why didn't he know why these things happen?

"That's where faith comes in."

"How do you expect me to have faith when I look into his face?"

"Faith isn't a magic carpet ride over life's problems. It is more of a bridge from island to island."

In the fifteen weeks of Justin's illness, Cindy and Rob walked the most painful journey known to mankind, of having to let go of a child. Even the best medical minds on earth, who find miracles to help so many, did not have one to make our Justin well again. It was March 29, 2001, shortly after his twelfth birthday, as he lay in Cindy's arms, that he passed on to heaven.

And then I knew.

God wanted you now and it was He that set you free.

19

Living Again

They say that heroism is to survive the experience without being ruined by it.

We go on because we believe. We believe that those whom we have loved and lost are in a better place; they are with God. We are comforted by a profusion of love, that which we give others and that which is given to us. Although we suffered pain and profound sorrow, we try to focus on the good things that were created along the way: a deeper love for each other, absolute clarity about our priorities, and a new closeness to God.

The paradox is this: those experiences that seemed greater than one heart could possibly bear are also the lessons of greatest value. My passage through stormy waters produced a true respect for the days and months and years that have been given back to me. I do not take my health for granted; I am aware of it every single day. I have a stronger bond with my belief system for I have felt the power of prayer. I am resolute about my values: Rich and our family are first; there is no compromise.

I try to know the people I care about more completely, on their terms, in their own unique and beautiful way, and to be unguarded and open so that they can know me better. My goal now is to influence the lives of our children's children so that there is some of me in their future. My legacy to them is the knowledge that now is the right time to experience love and joy, laughter and pleasure, despite how insurmountable our problems may seem. I want them to have strong values and not to waste time on a quest for happiness with things that are meaningless. Life is, after all, too short.

It is not my intention to explain these illnesses, for I hardly understand them myself. What I do understand is that cancer robs the world of enormous human potential and that is the shame of it.

Since my journey, I have become involved with cancer care organizations that seek to improve the quality of life for both patients and their families. Time and again, I have seen people regain control of their lives by approaching their illness with optimism, learning ways of coping regardless of their prognosis. These basic principles have been applied to cases of cancer of different kinds, in various stages, and with dissimilar conditions and, for the most part, have proved effective in making life better. Some experience fantastic results; with others the benefit is subtle. As treatments improve, more and more patients are being treated on an outpatient basis, shifting the job of maintaining a supportive environment to the home. Friends and family are often placed in the role of caregivers without training or tools and at times are ill-equipped for the daunting demands of caring for someone they love who is desperately ill.

My journey has caused me to think differently about cancer and I see it now as our social responsibility. We must become activists in fighting it, first through early detection and further by expanding our support of cancer services and research. We must be cognizant of the issues surrounding a healthier lifestyle as we make thousands of daily decisions that affect our environment, from chemical additives to the pollution of our natural resources. By becoming involved, we can communicate our outrage at losing over five million people yearly to cancer and influence political agendas that support solving the cancer problem.

Perhaps painful things happen so that we can more clearly see the value and significance of the events that make up our lives.

Perhaps they happen to temper us for the events yet ahead. I do not believe that they happen only to bring us closer to our faith, but that by coming closer to faith, we are better able to deal with the events.

Perhaps my purpose for surviving cancer was to share a conviction that there can be good in our world even during disasters. The key for us was to first be spiritually connected to each other and to God, giving us hope even during the darkest times. We trusted the scientific approach to therapy, but we also believed in the power of the mind to affect the body. Most importantly, we had an abundance of love.

Rich and I were already devoted to each other and deeply in love and I did not think that my relationship with him could have gotten stronger, but it did. When I was ill, he never showed me his fear and I know that he refused to accept that I might die. His incredible love gave me strength I did not know I had. He seemed always to know when I needed to laugh and when I needed to cry. The experience projected us into a new dimension that would not have been possible before. Now, we are one, in the inmost reaches of our hearts.

Perhaps the reason I survived is because I had not yet found the way to adequately express how very much I love him.

EPILOGUE:

From My Journal,
November 2000

We finally arrived in Milan after traveling all night and then spent the next day crossing the breadth of Northern Italy just south of the Alps by train, finally reaching the Adriatic Sea late that evening. We were exhausted by the time we retrieved our luggage in the pouring rain, hardly aware that we had at last reached our destination: Venice.

The line for passage via the public boat-bus was incredibly long and just as we were sure we would collapse at this final point of embarkation, a group of Venetians offered to share their gondola. As we squeezed in together, I noticed that they were quite well dressed, as though celebrating some special occasion.

"Oh, this is a very special day of tribute," the young woman spoke in flawless English, interpreting my observation to the rest in her party who all nodded in agreement. "For some it is to ask to be healed and, for others, to thank the Virgin for making them well. We go to La Salute, the basilica built to honor Her for saving the city from the plague in the eighteenth century. In English it is called the Church of Health." She then turned to her companions and spoke animatedly of someone's miraculous recovery and the tribute she was there to make for him.

I had thought that this trip, which seemed to terminate at the end of the earth, symbolized the end of the cycle of my illness. Then, it occurred to me that I was there, not as an ending but as a new beginning, a beginning that *was to start by giving thanks for the life I have and the many gifts it has given me, realizing for the first time that my illness was not a curse but a passage on my own unique journey.*

I knew little of Venice, conceiving it only as a mystical backdrop of novels, operas, and romantic films. I knew little of her history or her heritage and I had begun to question whether the long voyage was warranted. Then— slowly—as though lifting a giant velvet curtain inch by inch, this surreal city unveiled for us her majestic beauty, revealing architectural and artistic treasures created by a thousand years of meaningful expression. We were enchanted as we passed row after row of Renaissance palazzos and, captivated by man's attempts to carve immortality into stone, somehow we forgot the ache in our old bones.

On the first morning, I watched the sun rise out of the sea as the sleeping city awakened to meet the day. I could hear the sound of voices drifting up to our apartment as children and shop owners began the routines that defined their lives. The city had a kind of cosmic rhythm, like the waves washing up onto the shore and flowing back again. And, I wondered which of the children would pass on to their children the art and skill of their parents, just as their ancestors had done for centuries, generation after generation.

Believing that the chance meeting of the previous night was no coincidence, we agreed that we must go to La Salute before touring the galleries and museums. As we entered the basilica, I was instantly moved by the calm, serene surroundings, filled with the feeling that it was very holy there. As my throat began to close from the swelling emotion, I said a prayer and lit a candle, asking nothing for myself but help for those who are ill and suffering.

After a few days, we drove to Tuscany to spend a week in a small villa in the country. Again it rained, a hard, drenching rain, soaking the narrow roads and everything else along the way. Stopping for gas, we remarked about the bad weather conditions to the man from the village who was helping us.

"How can we be sad?" he laughed as he looked across the vineyards and olive groves being prepared for hibernation. "Do you see how thirsty is the earth? First we take off the old, and then we give her to drink. From this

comes new life, no?"

"Yes."

How appropriate that we had come here in the fall, when the cycle of life was so exquisitely illustrated.

We arrived that evening at the home of the proprietress of the villa we rented and were to be led to the property by her housekeeper, an ancient woman still in the proud employment of the landowner.

"Will you ride in the car?" I invited her in broken Italian.

"No, no!" she said as though the notion were preposterous, that getting in a car to ride through town and along a winding road was a waste of time and gasoline. "No," she repeated as she began the same walk as she had done for (what?) a hundred years? This great-grandmotherly woman shuffled down the road and I, of course, accompanied her while Rich drove quite slowly behind us. She was very proud to be the time-honored host of this old family property. As we walked and she talked, I looked into her face and observed an openness and kindness, a satisfaction with her simple ways and an honest pride in her existence. And, I could see with new clarity the beauty within a life well lived, for hers was a nobility of tradition.

This morning, I arose when the sun shone through the curtains as golden hues danced across the wooden floor, a warm autumn breeze blowing through the window. We have no specific schedule today and we will have none tomorrow. That's what it is like here and one of the reasons we chose this place. It is to be part of the balance we work to maintain in our lives now that I am well again.

Although it is still morning, I have been awake for hours and very, very busy . . . busy watching the countryside unfold as the sun pushes through the rain clouds and burns the morning into submission. Busy reading a book, watching the fog roll off the vines. Busy writing in my journal. Busy waiting for Rich to awaken to this amazing day. Busy.

Then, like stepping into a dream as I write, I recall my previous life and remember how easily one becomes caught up in the challenge of living and ends up desensitized to simple things. I know; we were there. But, not anymore. We came here to this remote place to hear the morning song of a rooster, to see the golden clouds of afternoon, to smell the crisp autumn air of evening.

And I wonder—as I wander—what purpose there is for me to discover in this life with this new gift of mine.

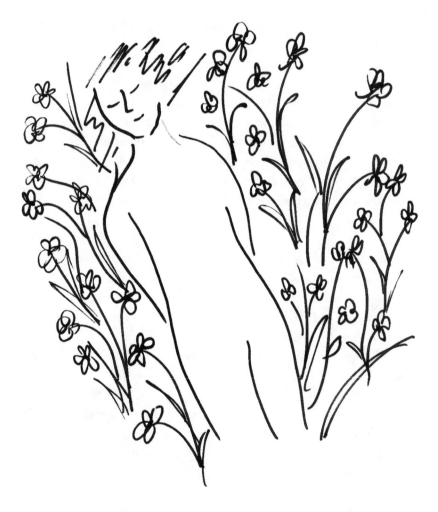

* * * * *

Today, there are over nine million Americans living with a cancer history. My purpose in sharing this very personal triumph is to help anyone who may be inspired to make his or her life better during this illness. Fortunately, we live in a time when medical break-throughs are happening at an incredibly fast rate, and soon there will be new therapies that will not burden the patient as did the old treatments. One day, finally, we will cure the disease. Until then, too many people will struggle to find a way to cope with it. This is one way—the way that worked for me.

* * * * *

Recommendations

There are many potential strategies presented in my story. I strongly recommend discussing any or all of them with your medical specialist and pursuing those suitable to your situation. There are, however, some points that I believe apply to anyone diagnosed with cancer.

1. **Give yourself a chance.** I still believe that the very best insurance is early and regular testing and examination. If you have a family history of cancer, get a thorough checkup. Do not assume that if you feel good, you are in good health. Do not delay if you are suspicious about symptoms. Time is the enemy that never sleeps, the killer cells reproducing day and night at an alarming rate. Of this I am certain: the earlier cancer is detected, the better the chances of survival.

2. **Treat your mental wellness as well as your physical wellness.** There are few things in life as frightening as a potentially fatal disease. Get help in dealing with the emotions that come with the illness, whether from a spiritual leader or therapist, prefer-

ably someone who is trained to deal with psychological distress of this magnitude. Professional services are available through many health care plans, hospital advocacy programs, or charitable organizations devoted to helping those diagnosed with cancer.

3.   **Get a nutritional plan.** Find a nutritionist or dietitian to help prepare a food plan that you and your helpers can follow. My plan evolved over time as we discovered how foods affected me. It is presented here for illustrative purposes only. Many HMOs offer nutritional counseling and may suggest diets to support your treatment. There are also community services that offer oncology–supportive diet evaluations and recommendations. *Be sure your doctor approves any nutritional or biochemical plan you consider using.*

4.   **Get an exercise plan that is appropriate for your condition.** Several health plans and fitness gyms that are willing to help cancer patients devise a plan to improve their strength during cancer treatment at no cost. Ask your local health club for professionals who are qualified to work with your specific medical condition. Cancer support organizations can offer nutritional and physical exercise evaluations and recommendations, including referrals to other qualified, legitimate resources.

5.   **Keep asking questions until you understand.** Most important medical information is relayed in technical terms that are unfamiliar to us. It is imperative that you understand what is being discussed about you or your loved one. If explanations are not clear, keep asking, even demanding until you understand precisely what is happening and what your options are. Do not be intimidated because of

your lack of knowledge; the most important thing is that you understand.

6. **Get organized.** Many illnesses such as cancer can be protracted over long periods of time. Having all pertinent information in one place is not only useful for daily management, but in an emergency it is invaluable. Notes, logs of events, names and dates of procedures, and questions for different specialists are referred to all the time. Do not assume that everyone involved with your case has a record of other procedures. Keep a journal.

7. **Understand and use your Patient's Rights.** Most hospitals provide them with admittance but patients pay as much attention to them as we do to the emergency evacuation maps in hotels. Voice your concerns about any person or procedure that does not seem right. Hospitals encourage patients to escalate problems so that they can remedy a bad situation before it becomes worse. The hospital administrators we dealt with were very supportive of the concerns we brought to their attention.

8. **Laugh whenever you can.** Everyone knows that to be diagnosed with this illness is horrible. But, living for months in a state of depression not only feels awful; it becomes a burden to those around you. Cut yourself some slack and have some levity. It will also accelerate your recovery.

9. **Never lose your dignity.** You are a whole person with the right and the opportunity to enjoy the best quality of life possible, regardless of your diagnosis.

10. **Believe.** And if you lose your faith, find it again. It is a wonderful companion in life and the hereafter. Simply open your heart.

Special Thanks

There are many people who must be thanked for their support during and the subsequent telling of our story. Their abundant knowledge, support, and faith became catalysts in my healing. They gave me the will to live.

In addition to those named in the book, many friends surrounded us with every imaginable kind of support and had a profound impact on my ability to move forward. In addition, Rich's friends knew that the focus is seldom on the caregiver and they supported him with care and concern.

I was lucky to have found competent and talented medical professionals. Dr. Kim R. Swartz, M.D., F.A.C.S. should be recognized for performing a successful Whipple procedure, which is not a universal skill. Dr. Paul Tseng, although driven by cutting edge medical modalities, was supportive of our holistic strategy and receptive to our theories about diet and exercise. Dr. David Van Sickle, M.D. placed the voice of his patient above all else. Finally, the oncology nurses at Northwest Cancer Specialists demonstrated extraordinary skill and compassion and I began to think of them as angels.

Dennis Milholm, Licensed Professional Counselor with the Association of Counseling Excellence, persuaded me to write my story and helped me find the freedom to hold nothing back. It was he who helped me see my illness as a gift that gave me a new sense of purpose of helping those embarking on their own journey, while imparting to me new clarity about love and life.

It was Joanne Leyva who first pulled me from the depths of illness to take charge of my own recovery and her knowledge and spirit that formed the foundation for the plan we followed. She was invaluable in the writing and remembering of the story.

Jim Harris, Paragon Media, convinced me that ours was a story worth telling and then helped me find my voice. He and Charlotte Harris, my editor at Skyward Publishing, have provided constant coaching and infinite patience.

Our family and friends gave me the hunger for good times yet ahead. And, as I imagine our grandchildren, nine at this writing, fishing off our deck with Papa Richie or making crafts with me, I must thank them for the hope that is reflected in a child's eyes.

My devoted husband, Rich, is still and always will be the essence of my soul. Each time I look at him, I am reminded that these times together were what I refused to give up. I thank him for making me want more memories of my lover and partner, my very best friend and biggest fan.

And I know there is a God for I am truly blessed.

My life was an illusion
   Before you came my way;
Was there anymore to life,
   I wondered everyday.
Then, there you were before me
   My dream fulfilled at last.
And magically the years and tears
   Dropped back into the past.
No more endless searching
   For what is really true.
For finally I am complete—
   I am a part of you.
You are my air and I am yours.
   We never really part.
We are one life for evermore,
   One soul, one mind, one heart.